Yang Deficiency – Get Your Fire Burning Again!

JONATHAN CLOGSTOUN-WILLMOTT

Frame of Mind Publishing
Edinburgh, Scotland, Great Britain

Contents

Introduction

Introduction request

First, when you have read this book, may I ask you to review it?

This will help others decide if they might benefit from it. Please post your opinion on Amazon or anywhere else you think would reach prospective readers. Of course I hope you will write a positive or at least constructive opinion!

However, if you have major reservations or criticisms, do let me know! Then I can improve the book for the next readers. Reach me through my website http://www.acupuncture-points.org, where on many pages there is a way to communicate with me. Thank you!

This book ...

This book is an elaboration of one of the most visited pages on my website. It covers the same ground as that page, but in much more detail and it takes the concept of yang deficiency much further, indeed out into life in general.

The book is in two parts. The first thirteen chapters are about the physical and mental sides experienced by individuals, with practical suggestions for self-help. From chapter fourteen onwards the emphasis moves to the world, the countries and their politics that we inhabit.

Because yin and yang encompass everything in the universe, yang deficiency can be looked at in many ways. So there is bound to be an element of repetition in some chapters which, although focusing on different aspects, start from the same basic theory.

Yang has many, indeed an infinite number, of ways to manifest:

- the flap of the butterfly's wing that supposedly influences the weather 10,000 miles away, an idea that one can easily conceive of
- the brute energy of a star such as the sun
- the political idea that changes a nation
- the question, or the unexpected right hook, that floors an opponent
- the transforming beam of an infant's smile
- the emotional flare-up in the heat of the moment
- the human spirit rising to the occasion
- the effects of libido at puberty
- the pull on the fishing-line that tells that you've hooked something
- the ability to decide

Chinese thought placed yang in the heavens above us, with yin below, the earth. Mankind stands on one but is inspired by and strives towards the other. We link them through our lives, and a successful life moulds them together. When we die, they separate, the body to the earth, the spirit perhaps carried on in the example we have set, the inspiration we have provided, the warmth for which we are remembered and, perhaps, in a greater group-mind potential.

Yin and yang carry no moral baggage. One can think of individuals who made a huge impression on their people, inspiring them to war and destruction, in hindsight remembered with horror. Yang creates, but also destroys and terminates.

Most of us think we are yang deficient as some point in our lives, even if temporarily, but we are often wrong! We may actually be suffering from either Qi Stagnation or Excess Yin, but not from yang deficiency.

Qi Stagnation[1] happens to everyone from time to time: a huge subject, I even wrote a book about it, the stress it engenders and what you can do about it. Stagnant Qi means things don't move and often you feel powerless, not from yang deficiency but because of obstacles: it produces all sorts of symptoms which, unless cleared, can lead to long-term incapacitating states of health, including tiredness. That tiredness can be mistaken for Yang deficiency.

Excess Yin is explained below. From the Chinese medical point of view, it has to be 'cleared' before yang can manifest properly again. Clearing the yin excess may be all that is needed for our yang energy to flourish again.

This is – obviously – only my understanding and interpretation of yang deficiency. There are other examples, but the book is long enough already!

Because the I Ching, the Book of Change, has been such a huge influence on Chinese thinking, I have included two examples of how it explains the possible outcomes of two very different situations, both with an element of yang deficiency. The first example is from when I used it to help me understand the possible forces at work during Britain's first referendum on British membership of what is now the European Union. The second illustrates some of the potential outcomes of a terrorist atrocity in the making, using a recent film as a basis.

1. http://www.acupuncture-points.org/qi-stagnation.html

PART I

THE INDIVIDUAL CONTEXT

CHAPTER 1

Yin and Yang types

An old way to classify personalities was into four types:

- Choleric: these people might nowadays be described as Type A people. They are competitive, pushy, demanding: only interested in people, including 'friends', for how they can help the individual look good or benefit his business or career. Outward-looking and upward-moving.

- Melancholic: these people are emotional, self-critical and interested in values: careful when making friends and easily hurt. Inward-looking and tend to be slightly depressive.

- Phlegmatic: these people are hard-working, steady, often non-competitive, with a sense of humour: friendly and less easy to hurt. Practical and undemanding, tending to look inwards. Can be stubborn.

- Sanguine: these people are positive and open, encouraging and friendly. Outward-looking. Not always hard-working.

Even nowadays, with all our insights and psychological knowledge, these four types and their attributes are easy to spot. With experience we can see that people are often a combination of types, say a sanguine-choleric, or phlegmatic-sanguine.

Usually one mode predominates. Since Jung gave us the concepts of introversion and extroversion, we realise that each type has several nuanced sub-types.

Indeed, Jung's work took the four main types and refined them, giving them slightly different meanings.

Balanced people can display any of these 'types' of personality according to need. For example, when first meeting people, being quickly able to get on the same wavelength as the stranger can make a huge difference to how the relationship develops. Whereas if you assume everyone is your own type and behave accordingly, you may put off 75% of people who aren't of your type.

Later, as you get down to work with your new colleague, displaying a phlegmatic attitude to getting through it makes it easier than being choleric about it. But if you definitely need to push something through obstacles, your choleric 'face' is needed. Later you may enter the melancholic mode as you consider all the options and refine how you might proceed in future.

Of these, the more yang-types are the choleric and the sanguine. The more yin-types are the melancholic and phlegmatic.

There is nothing good or bad in itself about these types. Each has merits and we all benefit from their strengths. The choleric needs the phlegmatic to get on with the job; the sanguine needs the melancholic's ability to research and think things through.

So it is with yin and yang types. If everyone were a yang type, there would be no stability, plans would be forever changing, and probably very little would get done.

On the other hand, if we were all yin types, life would go on but at a rather dull level. Still, if all of us were yin, perhaps we wouldn't mind!

The point is this: if you are a typical melancholic you may well feel that you lack effective yang qualities and energy. Reading this book may help you become more balanced, but don't undervalue your feelings and intuitions. They make you the valuable person you are! By all means develop a more rounded approach, but don't try to become what you aren't.

In fact, if anything, it is the choleric and sanguine individuals who may, for reasons explained later, need help re-kindling their yang energy.

CHAPTER 2

What are the Tao, Yin and Yang?

Before explaining yang deficiency, you have to know what yang means. For that you must also know what yin means! Then you see how they make up the Tao.

All and everything make up the Tao. The ancient Chinese thought it was impossible to say much about the Tao. The Dao de Jing (the 'Book of the Way') by Laoze is a kind of mystical primer on how to live with it.

Easier, though still difficult, was a way to understand its workings by dividing the Tao into 'yin and yang'. Yin and yang describe the movement or change of the whole cosmos and of every conceivable part of it.

Yin is, more or less, what you can see and what has been achieved. Yang, more or less, is the energy behind or within yin and its potential.

For us, our physical bodies are yin, the places we live: they become tiresome when we are ill, old or in pain. The energy that maintains life in the body is yang. Too little yang, and you feel flat. Too much, and your friends complain that you are 'hyper'.

Everything in the theory of Chinese medicine boils down to yin and yang: how they interact, how one or the other grows stronger or weaker, and how to get them back to dynamic balance and health.

The Chinese symbols for yin and yang show that yin was represented as the shady side of a hill, yang as its sunny side.

For many, it takes a few minutes to think you've understood this, and the rest of your life to realise you haven't.

Yang can produce yin forms. Yin forms give birth to yang ideas and energies. Each contains the seeds of the other and when either reaches an extreme, or point of no return, it transforms into the other.

- Day (yang) follows night (yin) which becomes day again.
- In high latitudes, towards the poles, days in summer are longer that nights. This season is more yang. Conversely, winter has longer nights: more yin.

There are many kinds of yang.

- Qi, or energy (but 'energy' fails to convey properly the idea behind 'Qi')
- Heat
- Mental 'spirit'
- Motive force – although this cannot be applied without some element of yin

Yang deficiency can *seem* to occur in several ways:

- You catch a bug, say a cold, and feel shivery and cold as the disease gets a grip on your health
- You suddenly, or within a few hours, get really cold, perhaps from not wearing enough on a cold day, or from being exposed to unseasonably freezing weather

- Powerful state control and surveillance of its citizens makes you feel powerless to act
- As you convalesce from a disease you find your energy weak, you avoid cold situations and drafts or winds, and feel low and dispirited
- You are naturally a chilly person, who wears more than others, even on warm days
- Your sexual libido takes much longer to recover than usual, or you've lost it
- The more tired you are, the colder you get. For instance, in the evenings you crave warmth more than earlier in the day

These can all seem like a deficiency of yang, but in fact in Chinese medicine, the first two (when you get shivery during an illness, and you get a chill from exposure to cold) are not classified as yang deficiency but as an invasion by what is called either 'Wind-Cold[1]' or just 'Cold[2]'. Nevertheless, they show a comparatively deficient yang situation.

Neither of these first two would have happened if your yang energy had been strong enough to repel the 'invader'. Nevertheless, your yang energy might have been quite normal, and healthy – just not strong enough to defend you against too powerful an invader. In Chinese medicine, the first thing to do is to clear the Cold or Wind-Cold that has invaded your body. Later, if necessary, you strengthen the yang.

You can tell the first two are from Cold invasion because typically they come on quickly – within a short period of time, perhaps just a few hours – of the trigger.

Also, in the case of catching the bug, (invasion by Wind-Cold) they come on with sneezing, a headache, perhaps a sore throat, and the symptoms are intense. You may also feel alternately

1. http://www.acupuncture-points.org/wind-cold.html
2. http://www.acupuncture-points.org/cold.html

shivery then hot for a few minutes, before getting shivery again. Or different parts of your body suddenly feel cold then hot, as your body's yang forces by turns waver then rally in defence.

In the case of the coldness from exposure (Cold invasion), it comes on quickly either while exposed to the cold conditions or soon afterwards – again, within a few hours. And the feeling of cold makes your tense up, and possibly frightened for your life. You may not be able to stop shaking from the cold.

In both these examples, sitting for ten or twenty minutes in a very warm bath (yang) or steam room might solve the problem. If your body responds by beginning not just to feel warm again but to perspire, you may have helped it to get rid of the invader. You will then recover faster, though obviously you should keep warm and avoid cold foods and drinks until you feel better. After a few days, depending on your underlying health and resilience, you should have recovered.

The third situation, of powerful surveillance and control, puts yang energies at a disadvantage. This is always a 'temporary' situation from which yang energies eventually break out. To prevent this, the state increases its power and control. It usually does this by removing 'difficult' members of society from public view: either to prison, or worse. Unfortunately, such 'temporary' situations can last many years.

The others listed are examples of yang deficiency, mainly the subject of this book.

RULES FOR YIN AND YANG

As a way of trying to understand the Tao, yin and yang, the Chinese put forward basic proposals or 'rules' about how they observed yin and yang to act.

1/ Yin and Yang oppose one another

2/ They support one another
3/ They destroy each other
4/ In certain conditions they turn into one another.

Rules 1 and 2

The first two are easy to understand if you think of a coin: there would be no coin unless it had two sides, each opposing the other but representing an aspect of it and supporting the other side. One side represents and bestows the authority of the state or the Crown; the other side states the denomination, the value of the coin.

A yin-like situation such as the lot of a disadvantaged, ill or forlorn set of people encourages someone to suggest ways for change. This leads to a visionary (yang) who inspires others to set up a company or charity or government department to change the status quo.

Eventually funds are found or grants extracted from government to initiate the enterprise. Willing volunteers assist.

As time goes on, the enterprise if successful grows and able administrators are found to run it, requiring salaries and pensions, for which more 'core' funding is necessary.

As the reach of the organisation increases, so does its core grow. Here the Yin core supports the Yang reach.

Then its ability to change and adapt slows, because of conflicting demands on it internally and externally.

At some time in its development, its progenitor, its original yang-like inspiration, departs the scene, unable to tolerate the yin-like machinations and torpor: often the managers find themselves opposed to his or her ideas, which they consider too disruptive. Here Yin opposes Yang.

If it is a charity, it is most yang-like in its infancy, when inspiration and vision rule.

It becomes increasingly yin-like the more structures, committees, administrators and rules it is governed by.

In the end, the situation changes. Sometimes this occurs because a more adaptive organisation out-competes it, or because the underlying need alters, or because the rules under which it was set up make it no longer appropriate. For example, churches are often gifted properties in the wills of parishioners. These properties come with tight covenants so that they can be used only for one purpose, such as to house the needy, and cannot be sold. Yet circumstances change, making what seemed like a wonderful gift an onerous burden, too costly to maintain yet impossible to sell.

Here the yang individual who set it up eventually loses patience and is opposed by the yin form he constructed.

Rule 3

The third rule is easy to understand.

- How a volcanic eruption (yang) can destroy a long-established city (yin) or more, as when Vesuvius erupted in AD79 destroying Pompeii;

- When a totalitarian state (yin) crushes its opposition (yang);

- When a Victorian family (yin) insists on its children (yang) being seen but not heard, thereby crushing the spirit of some of the children;

- When the Bolsheviks (yang) destroyed the Russian Tsarist constitution (yin) in 1917;

- As when voices of yang across the world destroyed Russian-style communism (yin) and the Berlin Wall came down in a few hours (yang).

Rule 4

This rule explains how coal can turn into energy: sunlight, absorbed by plants millions of years ago, gets compressed into a hard black substance that, after a lot of hard work, can be turned back into light. The same can be said of nuclear fusion and fission.

Good mediators can stop two opposing parties from destroying one another and create something new from the remnants of the old.

This fourth 'rule' is the one most people are interested in, although really we need to learn more about how to maintain civilisation by keeping the first two rules in a kind of dynamic tension without either ever becoming excessive to the point where the fourth rule takes over, let alone the third rule.

That means that individuals, families, communities, societies and countries have to learn to balance the books, to care for the less able or weak, yet allow for change, drama and excitement.

Unfortunately, that does not make for a completely stable situation, nor a comfortable one. It means that, for real health, there should always be allowance for yang energy to disrupt the yin. This view is not well-tolerated by those of a yin disposition.

It may mean allowing for disagreement, acknowledging the need for energy release through rash behaviour, even accident; for a black market; for even the odd crime; permitting the non-compliant or extraordinary – those who don't fit in, to flourish – to some extent!

(... But the 'rules' of yin and yang say that even such a society, if it ever became too settled, would contain the seeds of its own destruction. There is always a joker in the pack!)

Competition and Adversity

Another way to enable change by using the parameters of yin

and yang is that of competition. If competition follows certain rules (which are themselves subject to periodical review) and a society accepts this, then disruption and destruction may be reduced, or at least contained. The problem is that strongly yin-focused organisations often dislike competition, because it exposes weakness and hence inequality, for them uncomfortable conditions. However, the rules of yin and yang suggest that any organisation or country that suppresses change for long eventually has a very uncomfortable awakening, often followed by a great deal of suffering.

However much we would like things to continue as they are, to suit us, they will not. Some act of change or destruction, whether of a dictator, warlord, act of God or change of circumstances including death, will always occur in the end.

Yang deficiency never continues for ever.

Birth and Death

The final assertion of yang change is the act of dying, in its own way as yang a process as that of being born. At death, the old or former situation ceases. Then comes a process of destruction, quick or slow as the former body is picked to pieces. Eventually a new form replaces it as a new yang life emerges and takes yin form.

So a deficient yang situation occurs in a number of ways:

- When yin becomes overwhelming, for example ...
- When a powerful yin state begins to suffocate yang[3]
- When yin seeks to destroy yang energies

3. "Let the ruling classes tremble at a Communistic revolution. The proletarians have nothing to lose but their chains. They have a world to win. WORKING MEN OF ALL COUNTRIES, UNITE!"(From the final page of Samuel Moore's translation of the Manifesto by Marx and Engels.)

- When yin becomes extreme, either too powerful, too old, too inflexible, too unforgiving

- Or when yang becomes exhausted or dispirited

These help us to understand how to deal with deficient yang:
1/ Reduce opposition from yin
2/ Encourage support from yin
3/ Try to avoid situations where yin destroys yang, for as long as possible at least
4/ Marvel when yin becomes yang, and finally
5/ Use yang to increase yang
This book explores how to do this.

TAO, YIN/YANG IN MORE DEPTH

One way to acquire the rudiments of wisdom is to absorb the ideas behind yin and yang.

Yin is substantial, which means it has substance: it exists and you can often see it or touch it. It is easy to describe. At any rate, yin is usually much more substantial and long-lasting than yang.

The Pink Elephant

Think of it this way. It is quick and easy to conceive of something – a pink elephant, say. We can imagine things easily, even impossible things, like you see in the advertisements, or a pink elephant.

It might take another act of creation to produce in time the actuality of a real, live, healthy pink elephant or, if in your universe you already happen to have one, then a grey one as in mine.

But I am not the only person in this universe to be able to conceive of a pink elephant, even though they don't exist. Apparently it is quite easy. Lots of us can do it. Obviously it would not be difficult, though certainly unkind and probably cruel, to paint a perfectly healthy normal grey elephant in pink paint, and so be able to claim you have a pink elephant, though even this might be more difficult than you think ... first catch your elephant.

But, back to the thesis. Ideas are easy for us to conjure, whether that of a pink elephant or of Maglev trains.

Maglev Trains

Maglev ("Magnetic Levitation") trains use a very yang form of energy to raise and propel them. Why so yang? It is invisible and changes polarity very quickly. But to produce it you must first have the raw materials, the knowledge of what to do with them and the means to do it, and enough labour or power actually to build the thing. Then you need the whole energy and concrete infrastructure to make it work. If successful, you have something that is virtually soundless, in the absence of air-friction can go at any speed – ie apparently of infinite power – and seems to run like magic.

The point is, to produce that yang quality, you need a huge investment. That huge investment is the yin aspect of the Maglev train.

Olympians

Or take an Olympic Games Gold winner, a superb athlete. Start with the right genes, for which go back a number of generations. Then choose the right upbringing, food, environment and education. Then, encouragement. After that, personality, dedication, discipline and training.

What have I left out? Time. The whole thing must culminate

just when the Olympic Games come rolling over the time horizon.

And then, comparatively speaking, the whole thing is accomplished in no time at all, usually no more than a very few hours, sometimes just seconds, of precise, applied effort.

We applaud those who achieve at this level. They are the few who managed to bind their wherewithal together in the right way at just the right moment for just long enough to win. It takes a huge effort, and not just from the competitor, but from all the different parties without whose encouragement, experience and support the deed could not have been done. Do not forget, also, the investment by the host country in the event that made it possible.

These very yang displays rely on huge investment of yin resources.

So it is easy to imagine a yang 'success', but it can require immense supplies of applied yin resources to make it happen in reality.

From these few examples, you can understand some of the ideas within the concept of yang:

• Easy to conceive, takes effort to achieve

• To achieve peak success, everything must work perfectly in harmony

• Display

• Acts fast: is usually of short duration compared to organic development

• Sudden

• Involves change, from the preceding situation

• Destroys previous conditions (think of old sporting records being broken, or of the effect of earthquakes)

Examples of yang in action

- Light
- Heat
- Lightning
- A bomb – Explosions
- An accident
- Acts of vandalism
- Things that happen rapidly or suddenly: unpredictable
- Something which changes itself or situations fast
- Your imagination
- Initiative in action
- Independence of thought
- Revolutions or invaders that quickly destroy or usurp the status quo
- The act of procreation

However, although this is usually the way things work, sometimes what seems a small amount of yang rightly applied can wreak havoc or shift opinions or mountains.

Man has learned to harness yang to make life easy. The computer I type these words on and the light which helps me see the screen work via electricity, which, except when it sparks, I cannot see. But actually you cannot harness yang. You can, however, manufacture yin devices that produce yang. This takes a lot of resources, effort and time, all of them yin words. So we need yin to produce yang.

Or do we?!

The people who invented this yin-yang idea seemed to think that yang came first: if you like, that the thought preceded the action. It is currently believed that the universe began with a yang event, a big bang. This then created yin, and the fact that it then took over 14 billion years to produce the body you inhabit is testament to yin having to do all the work.

You, with the right genes, resources, effort and time can win the Olympics.

We are fascinated by yang.

- Children, however old, are attracted by fireworks, displays, excitement, the theatre, new films, competitions, drama, colour, fashion, parties, charisma

- We like movement, the excitement of the circus or the fight

- We watch or listen to the news to find out what's new

- We are in awe of the display of raw power whether it is of suns being created or the ability to spend fortunes to create the 'perfect wedding'

- By association we follow the famous, celebrities, and to emulate them we buy the stuff they wear or promote:

- We are attracted to the stardust of celebrity or top achievers, whether they are athletes, pop-singers, Nobel prize-winners, famous novelists ... but also dictators and generals who change the world

- We like humour, it makes us laugh. If we already know the joke, it falls flat. Humour usually needs to be unpredictable. The sudden change in viewpoint is funny.

- Sadly, over the centuries many have been and, even now, some are still attracted to the heroism of war. Many terrorists who die by the suicide-bomb (yang destroys yin) believe themselves to be heroes.

- Belief systems, including religions, are comparatively yang, though the more entrenched in their beliefs they become, the more fixed in their dogma, the more administration and systems and buildings they acquire, the more they become yin-like. Huge efforts are then made to maintain and control their 'static' belief systems, to educate the people in the 'truth', sometimes even to force these beliefs on others. In Christianity there were the Crusades and the Jesuits. Islam too has many examples, some prominent while this book is being written, of one sect trying to force its beliefs on the rest of us and by destroying the old.

- Lies
- The Masterstroke
- The 'Moment of Truth' – The 'Truth that sets you Free'
- Independent, objective discoveries, whether from sole investigators or thinkers or from academia unsullied by group-think

Yin situations are existing and only slowly changing, like the seasons and the annual organic growth and decay of life. They are the status quo. Creating them originally may have entailed a yang process, but since then they have settled down to a more comfortable regularity.

Insubstantial but still yin-like

What about governments, local governments, limited liability or joint stock companies, partnerships and institutions? These are an interesting variation on the theme. You might think that, because they are insubstantial, they are yang-like. After all, you cannot touch a national or local government, a joint stock company, partnership or other institution, though you can certainly touch their property, such as the buildings they occupy, and the people who manage them.

They are yin-like because they become, after creation, relatively unchanging, stable factors on which we depend.

As they become more yin, in many such institutions you find officials are appointed through a family-like process, the next in line, the most senior, or the one to whom most is owed, but not always the most eligible or enterprising, because originality rocks the boat. People brought in to provide creative thinking seldom last long. This eventually leads to poor management and inefficiency, the heavy hand of bureaucracy, price controls, tariffs and regulations: only those who toe the line are given or retain power and position.

Such a country, as this stultifying process runs its course, becomes weaker. It pours more and more of its resources into maintaining the status quo, often by repression and the build-up of police forces or by supporting the weaker members of society, all at the price of the development of good business practices, competition, enterprise and the market, all of which require or must learn the ability to adapt to change quickly, or they perish.

Capitalism is more yang than socialism because it is risky. If it succeeds, the prize may be considerable – wealth, potentially for all. Socialism is more compassionate but needs ever more resources and money to maintain the status quo. By comparison, if a capitalist enterprise miscarries, only a discrete number of people lose their money as it fails.

From this one can see that if a state allows itself to become too capitalistic, it risks losing everything and causing poverty and worse for its citizens.

For example, one reason (though by no means the only one) that jogged Scotland into joining England and Wales in 1707 to form Great Britain ("United into One Kingdom by the Name of Great Britain") was that Scotland had invested a huge amount in a failed enterprise (the Darien scheme, an ill-founded attempt to set up a new 'Caledonia' in Latin America). Scotland went more or less bankrupt in the attempt, ruining many of its citizens.

The longer any status quo continues, the more complex it becomes – 'complexity' is a yin-type word. Usually this is because, within it, there arise consequences not originally envisaged, so exceptions and diversions are created to absorb them without jeopardizing the whole.

Yang actions produce consequences that are yin-like.

A tax system designed to bring everyone into equality is later found to penalise a group whose voices become important, so the tax system has to change, little by little, to accommodate the new. It becomes more complex and refined (yin words) with more and more impossible situations that take more and more accountants, lawyers and inspectors of tax to resolve. In effect, more and more yang energy goes into creating and sorting out more and more yin minutiae.

Eventually, the longer and more extreme the yin state becomes, the more likely becomes a yang change, of the Rule 4 kind (at the extreme, yin turns into yang or vice versa) or Rule 3 kind (they destroy one another). The greater or more unchanging the yin, the more devastating the (yang) change when it occurs.

For example:

- in the economy and stock-markets you get greater and greater debt and higher and higher stock market prices until suddenly, as in America, you get the stock-market crash of 2008;

- in Russia, communism continued until more and more different vectors led to its impossibility as it tried to adapt to the Western world, and finally the Berlin Wall fell;

- in China the stock market raced upwards until suddenly it tumbled 40% in a few days;

- in an Agatha Christie detective story, you get a more and more complex situation with more and more possible explanations until in the final chapter the story teller supplies the bigger picture, or the last words of the book explain all that came before;

- The French Revolution at the end of the 18th Century violently overthrew centuries of Royal control and prerogative. The motto associated with it that eventually became institutionalized – Liberty, Equality, Fraternity – was very yang-like and inspiring. Unfortunately, it has caused philosophers many problems: the words are really rather incompatible with one another unless carefully defined, and defining them definitely takes the shine off the concept;

- Great Britain originated in 1707 when Scotland joined England. In the 21st Century there are movements to assert individual nation-hoods again. If this happens, the time it takes to affect the severance of bonds is usually comparatively short compared with the length of time the status quo has existed;

- in 2016 a huge debate in the United Kingdom developed over whether Britain (being the United Kingdom and Northern Ireland) should leave the European Union (EU), which had been in existence since 1951 in one form or another and which they joined in 1973. The EU has since been growing gradually with the accession of additional European countries. Although the UK managed to change the terms of its membership so that the UK would not be part of further European political integration and would keep its own border controls, in 2016 there suddenly grew a huge movement in favour of leaving so as to assert Britain's right to control its future alone. The two main arguments concerned borders (prompted by concern over UK migration policy which is subject to EU law), and alarm over the growing size of the EU, with equal rights for all its citizens, including the right to work in and travel between any other EU country including the UK. Essentially these were reactions to the EU's status quo, its size and power. This can be seen as a yin state reaching a 'impossible' stage, at which point yang will emerge and define its own borders again. At the end of this chapter is an example of the author using the I Ching in 1971, before the first referendum on joining the EU.

Summary: Yang corrections happen fast. Yin changes happen slowly, through organic growth or gradual erosion.

The flow of energy

The Chinese theory of yin and yang says that Yang energy, which is characteristically more warm than cold, is attracted upwards, towards 'Heaven'.

If you wonder why yang is warm compared to yin, think of friction which occurs as yin things grate against each other, producing heat, whereas yin things left alone don't move and so grow cold. Volcanoes erupt when immense gravitational and tectonic movements create heat, melting rock and forcing it out – and up.

Yin energy sinks downwards, towards Earth. Like gravity, yin is what we expect and are comfortable with. Yang disrupts that process. But as in a civilised society, where the more entrepreneurial efforts in the form of profits go to pay for everything the state needs to do its business, in the body, the yang force keeps blood moving, holds us upright, sends clear energy upwards so that we think clearly and don't fall over.

Every second or so, your heart produces a heart-beat. That single 'small' comparatively yang process keeps the whole of your body alive, by pumping warm healthy blood to your extremities and back. Without this pulse, your body would grow cold and die. As you age, your heart becomes less efficient, you become more inclined to need time to react and think, and you get more breathless and slower to recover from getting tired.

On the other hand, when you are young and just old enough to run around, you are easily excited and amused, entranced by everything: it is all new to you. However, lacking a large body and its reserves, you soon tire and you need frequent rests.

Perhaps when you first see snow you rush out into it, heedless of the effect of cold. Your grandmother follows you more sedately, watching carefully as you prance around. Suddenly the effect of your exertions and the cold makes you tired and upset. Your grandmother carries you inside, gives you a little warm sustenance and lets you sleep. An hour later you are refreshed and rush outside again.

Contrast that with your grandmother who, if she gets cold may need some days to recover. Indeed, if she becomes seriously hypothermic, her health may be permanently damaged and she could die, if not at the time then later when she next gets cold.

You are young and yang, she is old and yin – she cannot adapt so easily as you, though she has more mass, more experience and more resources: all yin words.

CHAPTER 3

Spheres of Action of Yin and Yang

Over a period of time, the parts of the body and the actions of yin and yang have been worked out, much of it in effect through the theory, experience and practice of Chinese medicine.

By appreciating yin and yang you can learn the essentials of Chinese medicine in about 4 minutes. It then takes a good ten years to work out how to put it into good practice. Conversely, it takes about ten years to learn Western medicine, but – if you have a prescription pad handy – about 4 minutes to put it into practice. (I attribute this light-hearted comparison between Chinese and Western medicine to Dr John Shen who said something like it at a seminar in 1980.)

In our bodies yang is on the outside: yin inside. Our immune force is more yang. Our minds are more yang than our bodies. What keeps us warm, inspired and upright is yang; what nourishes, cools, enables us to rest and gives us physical strength is yin.

The front and inside are more yin than the back and outside. The lower part of your body is more yin, the upper part more yang. The sharp or hard bits used for attack or defence are more yang: the soft bits which maintain the ongoing processes are more yin.

Compared to each other:

Yin parts of the body and mind	Yang parts of the body and mind
Inside	Outside
Front	Back and side
Ongoing maintenance process	Immune force
Body	Mind
Lower parts	Upper parts
Nourishing, relaxing and recovery modes	Energising, warming and uplifting modes
Physical strength and endurance	Motivation and inspiration
Contracting	Stretching
Restraint, stabilisation	Stimulation
Decrease, decline	Increase, growth
Blood	Qi
Material basis or substrate	Vital *functions*

Other Yin associations	Other Yang associations
Silence	Speech
Receiving	Giving
Being controlled by others	Controlling others, taking decisions
Getting 'stuck' in life	Moving on, getting on, in the world
Inaction; waiting; organic growth	Action; initiating; sudden change
Inward orientation	Outward orientation

From the above you may begin to recognise what happens when yang is deficient.

Note: if you have knowledge of the earliest correspondences

in Chinese theory as between yin and yang, you will realise that I have omitted some of them such as the association of yang with 'older', father, and man; of yin, with 'younger', mother and woman. In part these demonstrated the important part that hierarchy and respect for elders played in Chinese society.

Identity

The first requirement of a new being or body or state is identity. We can then think of it as a distinct being. The identity, its most yang aspect – the 'I am' of the 'that I am', is defined by its borders or by its description, later by its airs and graces, its personality, culture and history. But first, it must have a border, or it will get swamped or confused with something else.

Yang energy is sent by a state, or your body, to maintain or defend its borders, the very first requirement for a government or body. Hence you get the big fist and the armed forces. Later, sometimes much later, it needs to maintain order within the state, hence the police, in non-violent conditions a more yin-like institution.

In a new-born child, the first 'healthy' thing a child can do is make a noise. The more noise, the more powerful the lungs. Not for nothing are the Lung energies, in Chinese medicine, mostly in charge of what in West Medicine is called the 'Immune' function. In Chinese medicine this is called the 'defensive' energy.

Anywhere there are borders with the 'other' comes under identity, including the skin and the gastro-intestinal tract, the lungs and the level of mental energy needed for 'separate-from-the-other'-ness.

Other areas that yang energy covers in individuals:

• name – both family name and forename

- (for a machine, the identification, serial or unit number: its price)
- distinguishing features, physical and mental (eg short, tall, hair colour, skin colour, disability, intelligence, acumen ...)
- gender, address
- accent and type of clothing worn
- where you grew up as it impinges on who you are (eg Yorkshire; Scotland; Panama)
- identity or passport number
- 'personality' – the impression you make
- 'friends' or groups to which you belong
- political inclinations
- level of fitness and energy
- sexual orientation

Some of these are yin factors – for example your background – but to the extent they represent how others see you, they are yang too.

As we increase in numbers, we seek ways to distinguish ourselves, and may defend ourselves vigorously even when we have what others regard as a 'problem', witness those who see themselves as victimised for any number of reasons and use their victim-hood as a weapon.

To the extent that we do what many others do, we can be classified (fairly or not) with general features ascribed to us such as our psychology, needs, inclinations, obsessions and so on.

For example, those who take endless selfies might be classified as 'narcissists'.

In which case, our yang attempt to differentiate ourselves, to seem different to others or special, puts us, with the others so classified, into a yin group state, possibly to be exploited: perhaps another example of rule 4 in action!

Trying to stand out from society without concrete achievements or substance (yin factors) to our name is like confetti thrown in the wind without a wedding to celebrate. It is quickly blown away and forgotten, if it was even noticed in the first place.

For a country, the equivalents might be:

- name, location, borders
- distinguishing features of the country's geography
- languages spoken
- race, colour, creeds, of the people commonly associated with the country
- identity and personality of its leaders
- currency
- ability to defend itself

Yang features on the mental level include:

- awareness
- ability to think ahead
- ability to forestall – contingency planning
- preparedness to name and shame others, to recognise potential enemies[1]
- ability to retaliate, to defend ourselves, to destroy as well as to create

---

1. In Great Britain in the 1930s, Winston Churchill was one of the few to draw attention to the impending dangers from Germany. He later became one of Britain's greatest war leaders: very yang.

CHAPTER 4

The I Ching - the Book of Change

This book is more about how yang manifests in the body than about how it manifests in the economy and body politic but the theory can be applied to any situation at all. Indeed, the classic book of Change, the I Ching, sets out a basic 4032 ways in which things may happen.

The I Ching is probably the oldest text in the world (BCE~750BCE) on the interplay between Yin and Yang.

To demonstrate one way the ancient Chinese dealt with the yang deficiency of indecision, here is what happened when I consulted the I Ching.

Using the I Ching in 1971. Indecision on the author's part was a form of yang deficiency

The question posed on 27/10/71: "Will Great Britain enter the Common Market within the next year and what circumstances are attendant on the matter?"

The method used to find which 'hexagrams' to consider was by 'throwing' the yarrow sticks. This 'throwing' is a careful procedure, in no way haphazard, taking perhaps 30 minutes although people get faster in time. Nowadays there are electronic methods of getting results, but the physical 'throwing' of the sticks induces a contemplative state of mind highly conducive to interpreting the outcome. Mathematically, it is apparently slightly different to using coins and, probably, getting a computer to generate the result.

The result was hexagram 44 with a 'moving' line in the fifth place, creating hexagram 50.

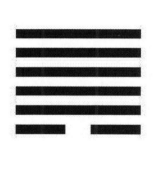

The above is hexagram 44. Its name, translated, means temptation, or allurement or encountering: the encountered situation meant is where there is potential danger for us. A strong other party (the texts say 'woman') may be too much for us.

(If you take umbrage at this use of the word 'woman', please consider that the texts consulted were written probably 2500 years ago in a culture very different from ours and where words often had several meanings different to those we are used to. Also, please consider that translation of these ancient ideas into modern English is subject to many hazards. However, that said, I think the texts were probably not written by women!)

At the time I took this to mean that we might never be completely happy about the relationship with the Common Market, nor give ourselves completely to it but that our feeling about it was that we felt very tempted to join. Also, secondarily, that because of the moving line, explained next, this relationship with the Common Market was able to change – and it was entirely our decision and within our power. By taking that decision, we demonstrated power which we could go on to use for the common benefit.

The fifth line (up from the bottom) is a 'moving' yang line, changing into a yin line. Interpretations since antiquity have suggested that this represents a ripe fruit, not necessarily obvious at first, but available in time for the taking.

I took this to mean that, because it is in a strong position (what is called a 'commanding' position, a reference to how the dynamics of the hexagram and this line's position work in practice) it was entirely up to us to take a positive role. Also, the 'ripe fruit' of the new relationship would manifest fully only in time.

Hexagram 50 is formed when the fifth line up from the bottom of hexagram 44 becomes a yin line.

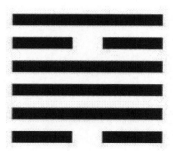

The name for this hexagram is much clearer: it is either a 'sacrificial vessel' or a 'cauldron' – a container with auspicious properties and potential.

The overall meaning to me at the time was that Great Britain was anxious about joining itself to what seemed like a very powerful yin energy; that it might never be completely in accord with this; that by joining we could, however, create something that could be much more than the sum of its parts, with great potential for all the peoples involved – and it was up to us to take that initiative.

The Benefits of Hindsight

Perhaps Britain did not take advantage of EU membership as fully as it might have. At any rate, in 2016, it voted to leave.

CHAPTER 5

Yang Deficiency Explained – Introduction, Mental and Physical Symptoms

In the greater sense, yang deficiency leads to a shortage of buzz, of excitement, of originality, and of colour. Without yang, life becomes more mundane, more normal and more reliable.

Without yang disturbances, it is easy to order one's life. The buses and trains run on time. People behave sensibly and predictably. The ill, disabled and weak are cared for. The young are encouraged and educated, their elders are supported, respected and eventually proceed to a calm pain-free death.

Everything is very civilised! The government defends the interests of the country and its inhabitants, raises the money to do it and everyone is happy.

Sadly, this yin-like status quo never lasts for long.

Someone always wants change. If there are too many bourgeoisie, that means there are workers who cannot break into that circle. There are always the jobless and the ill. There will always be immigrants and emigrants. There will always be trade adversaries who try to out-compete us, or someone who wants our fish, water, wealth or mountains. There are always voices crying out for change, whether it be to provide money and succour for the dispossessed, the starving, the disabled or the feckless; or to inspire us with new religious revelations. There is always someone seeking advantage who wants to go or to come, disturbing us.

Yang will always assert itself, eventually. Sometime it takes the form of the market, at other times it is the weather, or one of the seven deadly sins. I sit here, typing away comfortably then the telephone rings and a patient wants my attention, a yang energy disturbing my yin equilibrium. Then I sit typing again for a while, until I get hungry or run out of mental energy. Then I go off to give my creative juices time to refill: I take a rest (yin).

Soon afterwards, the yang energy reasserts itself and I sit down to write more for a while (yin) – until the next disturbance (yang) interferes or again I need a rest (yin) or a change (yang).

In our bodies, however, a yang deficiency can continue for some time.

How does yang become deficient?

- by lack of inspiration, passion, courage, warmth, desire, reactive speed, excitement, independence, humour, dynamism, decisiveness, clarity of thought, imagination or spirit
- by lack of yin resources to enable it to continue
- by being overwhelmed by yin forces. Yang forces against us tend to want to destroy us.
- by over-strain or overuse

How can it become strong again?

- by receiving the right amount of warmth, inspiration,

fervour, ardour or enthusiasm to re-ignite the yang passion, its 'spirit', (reinforcing yang)

- by getting enough time for it to recover through rest and nourishment (yin)
- by removal of adverse yin forces: reduction or removal of excess yin
- by desisting from overstrain and overuse

The rest of this book explores some of these themes.

However, there is yet another way in which yang can seem deficient. Often, because of circumstances, personality, frustration, illness not properly cured and other factors, including Qi stagnation, we seem to lose our joie de vivre – our yang 'drive'.

This can happen because of a build-up somewhere in our bodies of heat. This inflammatory situation may 'hide' from us for many years, appearing as mild irritations in our overall health.

In the long-term, it produces chronic diseases which wear us down. In the short term it may produce mild yang-type irritations that irk but do not stop us.

This situation tends to occur where symptoms have been suppressed, for example with strong medication, so that the underlying 'disease' has not been properly ejected from the body. Such an ejection or 'cure' usually only happens through an acute re-occurrence of the original disease.

For many of us this acute re-occurrence or re-expression of the disease is not a desirable solution, given that we sought to suppress the original manifestation of the disease, and had the means to do so.

Chronic examples include the following, the symptoms of which nowadays we can often mask with modern medication.

- Chronic Athlete's foot

- Skin eruptions, including eczema
- Sore joints that surgeons suggest we replace
- Sore, heavy, muscular stiffness or pain
- Nails that have ceased to grow properly
- Tooth/gum root canal infection
- Chronic burning pains, for example in the stomach – suppressed with antacids
- Chronic Reflux after eating
- Ongoing Constipation with dry stools
- Recurring Genito-urinary infections
- Tendency to harbour grudges
- Certain types of headache
- Chronic Lymph gland problems
- Dryness or heat anywhere, including eyes, red eye, blepharitis, floaters
- Occluded arteries or veins from plaque
- Where bones fuse together preventing movement

These kinds of examples tend to multiply with age. Eventually some can lead to tumours and cysts.

From where might these conditions originate?

- Many come from bad hygiene and poor nutrition – perhaps we eat foods that give us quick energy but lack real nutrition: that quick energy leaves waste products that our bodies cannot shift.
- Others may be 'enabled' through previous fevers which themselves might come from infection, osteomyelitis,

lymphoedema, drug medication, malignancies, inflammatory diseases etc. Some of these diseases can be caught from pets or via immuno-suppression.

- Poor breathing means we lack oxygen to 'burn' the waste products

- Not taking enough exercise means our bodies fail to circulate energy and blood, grow weak, and cannot 'burn off' toxins, including those caused by stress

- Poor fluid intake means our bodies cannot flush away waste products

Generally, these hot and inflammatory conditions if chronic may (eventually) drain the cooling, absorbing yin resources of the body. Without adequate yin, yang cannot flourish, lowering our energy and making it impossible to clear away the build-up of inflammatory toxins.

Like secret passions never admitted, these can eat at the soul and reduce the energy available for fun, joy, warmth and creativity. The body's yang has somehow become separated into two parts, one manifesting as the impediment, depleting the amount of energy available for the other.

Sometimes the ongoing cause is not drinking enough clean water over a long period of time. Water deficiency means inflammation cannot be cooled and washed away, so it festers.

Modern medicine is very good at controlling these underlying inflammations, so they tease and poison us inwardly, slowing us down: additionally, the medication itself produces unwanted side-effects that diminish us. It is as if so much of our body's energy goes into suppressing the symptoms or dealing with the chronic consequences that there is little creative yang left to inspire and change us.

There are therapies that aim to release this trapped heat.

They often require dedication and time but for those who navigate them, the effect on energy and life can be transformative.

However, (this is a 'plug' for acupuncture), some kinds of acupuncture appear to be able to reduce pain and inflammation for considerable periods of time without the need for a release through re-occurrence of the original or causative disease.

Trying to increase yang without first resolving these underlying chronic sources of inflammation can inadvertently increase the inflammation instead of the yang creativity.

MENTAL SYMPTOMS OF YANG DEFICIENCY

Very yang people are pushy, demanding, enterprising and often ebullient. They react fast to interference: they do not hang back. They have lots of ideas and can be exhausting for the rest of us. Manic people display many yang qualities.

So where there is a lack of yang, you get the opposite.

In a healthy individual, clear yang energy is sent upwards to nourish the brain, the sight, the hearing, the ability to smell and taste. You notice its lack when woken suddenly from deep sleep, when at first you feel woozy, possibly slightly dizzy, even confused, with sounds and odours making not much sense. As you adjust to being awake, your thoughts clear and your senses sharpen.

Typically, people very yang deficient appear:

- to lack confidence and initiative
- slow to respond
- hesitant to make up their minds
- tired or easily tired

- non-competitive
- reluctant to give you their opinions; prefer to remain quiet
- sometimes indifferent, even apathetic, as if from an unequal struggle with life
- weak to defend their 'corner', their interests, their future well-being
- indifferent or reluctant to play, as in sport, or social interaction, or wit or humour or games
- to need encouragement or support
- lacking interest in style, design, the why and how of things
- not interested in ideas
- to lack vision
- to be easily led

Bringing the mind to focus on topics can be hard. Collecting their thoughts is a sluggish process as they hunt for words, and they forget important arguments. When responding to you they do so hesitantly, even incorrectly, as if their senses are less reactive and slowed down. They don't grasp ideas quickly and can seem dull-witted.

If pushed or stressed, they make poor decisions, if they can decide at all.

Often they avoid contact with energetic, pushy people, tending to withdraw, to brood over their condition: depressed. It can be hard to get them to speak though occasionally you find yang deficient people who speak hastily, without thought (they are probably also yin deficient).

Often there is brain-fag. They are exhausted, lack will-power and cannot be roused to show enterprise or to organise themselves. In a way, they seem to have given up, listless, easily swayed by events. There may be a sense of hopelessness, and a fear of what life may bring.

But in the early stages, you may see little of all this, just someone who is tired out and apathetic, who stands up for himself with difficulty.

Working in mind-numbing circumstances, doing jobs that are uninspiring and over-controlled, or activities which lay you open to exploitation or abuse can also deplete your 'spirits'. In that case what happens depends on your yin resources and balance. To preserve health, you must first get enough regular rest. But eventually you need to take a yang action, to put up a barrier, or absent or separate yourself from the destructive forces.

For instance, a patient was a carer and counsellor for the mentally unstable. Long months of trying to resolve often impossible demands and of receiving abuse wore her down. Eventually her family persuaded her to seek medical help. Her doctor put her on sick leave and recommended medication, although in fact she sought acupuncture. The treatment mainly consisted of removing acupuncture channel blockages, then balancing yin and yang, then stimulating yang slightly more than yin (not least with humour and encouragement).

Once her spirits returned, she was able to return to work, albeit with changes in her work patterns which she had developed the strength of mind to demand of her employer.

Another patient, in her 70s, came for treatment because she had been diagnosed as having the early stages of Alzheimer's, a form of dementia. Her facial colour was grey, she looked tired and hopeless, with lined, shrunken facial skin. She said she was always cold. She neither smiled nor laughed, and her voice remained low and hesitant. She stood slightly bent, head lowered. I diagnosed yang deficiency, but also that she had some Blood Stasis, a history of considerable frustration and bad decisions, and Qi deficiency.

After the first treatment (to start to clear Blood stasis, to move her Qi, to stimulate Qi and Blood and with moxibustion[1] and laughter to raise her spirits, her face filled out, her facial colour improved enormously – in fact she almost looked flushed – she stood better, her conversation was normal, and she laughed easily. The spark in her eyes was rekindled and she looked forward to the next treatment.

Did I think that I had 'cured' her Alzheimer's? Certainly not, but I knew her yang energy was stronger, in much better balance with her yin. With more balance between her yin and yang, I would expect her Alzheimer's to develop only slowly. However, I also knew that she would need occasional ongoing treatment.

PHYSICAL SIGNS OF YANG DEFICIENCY

Since Yang represents the active form of energy, when yang is deficient you get signs of inactivity and tiredness.

In the body, the yang acupuncture channels all go to the head, and all of them except one (the Stomach channel) cover the sides and back of the body.

These are the areas that, if attacked, we turn to our assailant, by running away (when we turn our backs), by hunching up into a ball, or by hitting or kicking with the yang surfaces of the hand, elbow, leg or foot – and the head-butt!

The following is an elaborated version of the traditional symptom list usually described in Traditional Chinese medicine texts.

Yang deficiency shows up as a tendency to allow others to trample on us, to produce physical signs of the 'giving in' we display mentally.

What do you see if someone has given in?

1. Moxibustion uses the leaves of a plant, Chinese mugwort, artemesia chinensis. These burn slowly and steadily and can be used safely to warm the body or acupuncture needles inserted to stimulate yang energy. See also http://www.acupuncture-points.org/moxibustion.htm

- They stoop or hang their heads – their posture 'deflates'
- They look down or away from more confident people. (Of course, do not confuse this with many cultures where it is deemed inappropriate for lesser ranks to look directly at their seniors. Likewise, in 'Western' cultures many women take care not to look strange men in the face if they wish to avoid an encounter.)
- They feel easily tired: fatigued
- They prefer to sit or rest
- They become quiet
- They move and react slowly
- They want to be cared for and nourished
- They usually like warm, gentle massage
- They like their scalp being stimulated or stroked (which helps to bring yang upwards)
- They usually like someone else to take responsibility
- They prefer warmth, both externally and in what they eat or drink: for some, this warmth takes the form of warming drugs, like alcohol
- They can be magnetised by appropriate encouragement, vision and exhortation, though many prefer to withdraw from life's hurly-burly
- Pallor: their facial colour is often white (or dark blue, even black, when there is weakness in Kidney energy)

Specifically, Chinese medicine has noticed that if this (yang deficiency) goes on for long, there follow physical symptoms which relate to the energy organs ('zang-fu[2]' organ) most affected, such as:

2. http://www.acupuncture-points.org/zang-fu.html

- Weakness, even debility, fatigue, including chronic fatigue syndrome

- Many such syndromes contain what Chinese medicine terms 'Damp[3]'.

- Susceptibility to mild infections like the common cold, with slow or difficulty recovery that often ends in some kind of chronic condition like sinusitis, otitis or pharyngitis, often signs of what Chinese medicine terms 'Phlegm[4]'.

- These conditions are often accompanied by swollen lymphatic glands round the neck or in the armpits or groin.

- Back pain, mainly lumbar, though can be in other areas of the back (If in another place, such as between the shoulder blades, this may confuse your acupuncturist – but too bad: let her work it out!)

- Autoimmune allergies or diseases

- A sense of pressure, which can be felt in the head (often the forehead, but can be on the vertex or at the back), or on the sternum, or in the eyes

- A sensation of what is called 'formication', (it feels like ants walking over your skin), on the scalp, spine or limbs (Note: formication can also be a sign in Chinese medicine of what is called 'Wind[5]', often from a deficiency of Blood, a form of yin)

- As yang may fail to reach the head properly, there may be postural vertigo, meaning that if you stand up too fast, you feel dizzy.

- Faintness or Fainting: if yang fails to bring blood to the head. This is worse for standing for too long or for walking slowly or carrying heavy things

3. http://www.acupuncture-points.org/damp.html
4. http://www.acupuncture-points.org/phlegm.html
5. http://www.acupuncture-points.org/wind.html

- The immune system may be slow to respond to new pathogens

- Without sufficient yang, bodies work less efficiently. Symptoms depend on where the yang deficiency is most marked, but the kinds of symptoms that yang deficiency people get include the following:

- Weight gain (because there is not enough yang, either intrinsically or from lack exercise, to burn up the food eaten and utilise stored fat)

- Water retention, oedema and problems with urination (see below)

- Feeling cold: for example, cold lumbar back, cold limbs, cold hands and feet

- Dislike of cold environments or of getting cold

- Urine: frequent and pale. In people worn down by disease or age, there may be incontinence. This symptom seems at variance with the symptom above of water retention. Both are possible: it depends on which zang-fu (or energy) organs are affected.

- Legs heavy and sore, especially knees

- Weakened connective tissue making the individual more easily injured and susceptible to ligamental weakness, with ptosis and and a tendency to prolapse of organs

- Respiratory: difficulty breathing, often wheezing

- Respiratory problems include what happens when fluids collect in the lungs and cannot be spat out. Overnight or over a period of time, sometimes from yin deficiency, these fluids gradually thicken until they form a plug. This can be very hard to expectorate and can lead on to bronchiectasis, where after persistent infections, the airways in the lungs widen, lose their elasticity and cannot expel pus. However, this is often a complicated condition and yang deficiency might be just one part of the diagnosis.

- Secretions increase (see below)

- May have a soft voice, even a weak voice, easily tired by speaking much, by arguing or by shouting or trying to sing loudly (this displays Lung qi deficiency)

- Bowel movements: often urgent on waking, (this is usually called 'daybreak diarrhoea') and the stools are moist, even wet, and loose, and can be diarrhoea. This is because the lack of yang means that the stools are not dried out: then on waking, the resultant liquid stools cannot be retained. With yang deficiency, these stools do not usually smell offensive.

- ... sometimes the opposite, when there is a lack of movement in the bowels. This is caused by the Kidney yang energy being unable to move the 'qi' and the bowels, so everything grinds to a halt. In this case the stools themselves may not be too dry, unless the condition is very chronic (dry stools are more common in yin deficiency[6], which itself can be caused over time by yang deficiency). This condition is more common among older people. If the stools have become so dry that it is impossible to move them, a practical solution is often a colon cleanse to get things started. Good massage on the abdomen and back helps. Exercise and the right diet are vital for ongoing bowel health.

- People can be exhausted by their bowel movements. The little energy they have is soon exhausted by straining for a movement.

- Bowel motions can be so loose that there is bowel incontinence

- Perspiration: during the day more than at night (night sweats have several causes, including from what is called food

6. http://www.acupuncture-points.org/yin-deficiency.html

retention[7], from fever and from yin deficiency) and is sometimes mainly on the head or forehead.

Men:

- Low libido
- Impotence: this can be either lack of desire and/or of the ability to produce and maintain an erection (though Blood is also needed, a yin resource)
- Spermatorrhoea
- Poor sperm quantity or health

Women:

- Low libido
- Leucorrhoea that is watery
- Sterility

Free Secretions

This means that, lacking a secure yang energy, the exterior is poorly guarded and things escape. This becomes more noticeable when the situation includes Qi[8] deficiency which it often does.

There is a saying in Chinese medicine that 'when Qi is weak, fluids leak'.

Secretions (ie fluids) include

- perspiration
- tears

7. http://www.acupuncture-points.org/food-retention.html
8. http://www.acupuncture-points.org/qi.html

- saliva
- stools
- urine, and
- nasal secretions.
- They also include Blood, which can mean easy nosebleeds or from haemorrhoids. (However, there are other reasons for both nosebleeds and bleeding haemorrhoids eg Heat[9] and syndromes such as Liver-Fire[10].)

For example, yang deficient people who are also qi deficient often find that their eyes stream involuntarily, they sweat much more than normal and they have more saliva than usual.

People who are partially yang deficient may have cold noses – so their noses drip in cold weather. This happens more as people age, when specific zang-fu or energy organs begin to lose their youthful vigour or yang, and signs of coldness accumulate.

Secretions due to Qi deficiency are usually clear and watery.

Yang deficiency will lead to the appearance of what seems like excess yin (because lacking yang, yin seems greater, for instance by the appearance of excess secretions), but as the condition continues, yang's deficiency will begin to drain yin resources too (just as a trail of fuel in the wake of a car suggests the fuel tank is leaking, and the car will shortly stop).

Of course, many diseases quickly exhaust yang, so some of these symptoms come as add-ons with or after other conditions or diseases.

With low levels of yang energy, the body may be slow or even resistant to treatment for any condition.

Treatment for some kinds of yang deficiency initially produce exacerbations or aggravations as the body cannot integrate the extra energy. This can be very disheartening.

9. http://www.acupuncture-points.org/Heat.html
10. http://www.acupuncture-points.org/liver-fire.html

Yang deficiency as it progresses

Yang deficiency affects mainly the following energy organs: Stomach[11], Spleen[12], Lungs[13], Heart[14] and Kidneys[15].

There is often upper body weakness, and poor breathing patterns, either a consequence or cause of poor posture. Of course, genes play a role, but by right example, teaching, exercise, diet and discipline good posture can be achieved. If the lungs and chest don't fill out properly when breathing, they become receptacles for Phlegm[16] (a yin phenomenon) inviting bronchial disease.

As the disease improves and the patient convalesces, to what extent yang deficiency symptoms continue depends on other factors, such as:

• Kidney essence or 'Jing-essence[17]'

• The health of this depends on your previous health and that of your parents when you were conceived.

• Your age. Younger people usually recover faster, having greater supplies of Jing-essence than their elders. However, a severe illness can drag them down a long way, so this does not always apply.

• How debilitating was the disease you've just had. The more severe it was, the more it drew on your Jing-essence resources, leaving less available for Yang.

• Whether the patient rests enough and observes sensible lifestyle habits until better. If he or she goes straight back to

11. http://www.acupuncture-points.org/stomach.html
12. http://www.acupuncture-points.org/spleen.html
13. http://www.acupuncture-points.org/lung-qi.html
14. http://www.acupuncture-points.org/heart.html
15. http://www.acupuncture-points.org/kidney-function.html
16. http://www.acupuncture-points.org/phlegm.html
17. http://www.acupuncture-points.org/jing-essence.html

an intense exercise or work schedule, one that over-strains or over-trains, yang will take longer to recover.

• Further exposure to cold is detrimental to yang recovery.

Pulse

The **pulse**[18] picture of yang deficient people is 'slow' and 'weak', and may be 'deep' or 'hidden', often quite hard to feel at the wrist. Or it may be discernible on one wrist but not the other. (In general, the left wrist pulses are more important. If only the pulses on the right wrist can be felt, treatment will take longer to succeed.)

What do these pulse diagnoses signify? In Chinese medicine, there are twenty-eight possible different pulse qualities, including fast and slow. Each has a different implication for health:

• Slow pulse: the slow pulse has a number of possible interpretations, one of which is invasion by Cold, another being yang deficiency

• Weak pulse: means deficiency of yang, qi and/or Blood

• Deep pulse: means either a strong battle between the body's defence forces and an invading force, or deficiency of yang qi and Blood

• Hidden pulse: likely to indicate an extreme case of yang deficiency. (The hidden pulse is hard to feel, being so deep.)

Tongue

The **tongue**[19] picture seen most often with yang deficiency is pale, swollen and moist:

• pale because of the body's inability to bring sufficient good-

18. http://www.acupuncture-points.org/pulse-diagnosis.html
19. **http://www.acupuncture-points.org/tongue-diagnosis.html**

quality Blood to the head (healthy yang energy rises upwards, bringing Blood with it)

- swollen because since the individual is yang deficient they are also qi deficient which means the fluids in the body lack movement, so pool there and

- moist because this is yang *deficiency*. Yang is drying, yin is moistening. In the absence of sufficient yang, yin-moisture remains and accumulates.

Pain

Yang deficient people don't usually suffer strong pain. If they do, it does not last for long.

Yang deficient pain is more a kind of dull, bruised soreness, or heaviness, or an ache, with coldness.

Commonly this is felt in the joints, if nowhere else. The first joint to feel it is often the knee, because yang deficiency usually means Kidney deficiency, and the Kidney energy has been noticed in Chinese medicine to have an affinity with the knees.

However, knee pain may also indicate weakness in Stomach and Spleen yang energies. The Stomach and Spleen acupuncture channels run down the front of the thigh and leg on either side of the knee-cap: very important for leg strength and resilience.

The heaviness can be anywhere.

- In the head, you see them hanging their head, or stooping, or resting it against something.

- The arms and/or legs just literally feel heavy. It is an effort to raise the arm or to stand up from sitting, let alone to climb stairs or a hill. If climbing, they may need frequent rests.

- However, part of this crosses over to being due to qi deficiency, which is often felt first in the anterior thigh muscles.

Pain due to yang deficiency improves:

- From rest
- From warmth
- From gentle massage
- From inspiration and excitement. Sometimes, raising the spirits is enough to clear the pain. In the first instalment (2010) of Sherlock Holmes with Benedict Cumberbatch and Martin Freeman, 'A Study in Pink', Watson when introduced is using a walking-stick/crutch after a painful war injury. He is clearly in low spirits. However, as the story develops, excitement grows and when the first chase starts he drops the crutch, never to need it again. One may speculate that in times past powerful leaders could inspire their followers so much that they forgot their ills.

Qi Deficiency

Being on the same spectrum, it is sometimes difficult to distinguish between yang and qi deficiency. In general, yang deficiency is a more extreme kind of qi deficiency but sometimes the symptoms are not what you might expect.

For example, it is possible for you to be qi deficient yet not have yang deficiency. Usually, the qi deficiency is quickly mended by good sleep and food. A yang deficiency, however, takes longer, and coldness, which is often present in yang deficiency, can exist even when there is no qi deficiency.

For example, the author of this book tends to be a little yang deficient, but usually has plenty of qi. This means that he is particularly sensitive to **cold** and easily made ill by it. Being yang deficient means that his Spleen yang is also weak, making it important that he avoids too much food that is regarded as being cold in nature, or damaging to his Spleen energy.

(Spleen-weakening foods are typically those that are raw, cold, uncooked, chilled or sweet – and also those which are difficult to digest or in too big a quantity. See also chapter 8 under Nutrition.)

Western Equivalents

Any disease that produces symptoms of coldness or tiredness is potentially showing signs of yang deficiency. Why 'potentially'?

'Full' conditions, also known as 'Excess[20]*'*

Because the disease may be what is called a 'full' disease. With this kind of disease, your body is in aggressive mode, which you experience as cold.

For instance, let us say you catch a cold virus – though the principle applies whether it is a virus or bacteria. You feel cold and your body may actually be a bit colder than usual, though often you may have a fever, even though in yourself you feel cold. The cold symptoms can give you strong shivering or shaking.

Here, the symptoms are temporary, while your body deals with the invader. Usually, being in a warm place and wearing warm clothes is not enough to make you warm up. Even sitting in a sauna or hot bath might not do it, unless you stayed there for a long time. Generally, your body needs to go through a process as its defensive forces muster and eventually overcome the trespasser. While this proceeds, you feel ill.

---

20. http://www.acupuncture-points.org/excess-or-deficient.html

Empty or Deficient conditions

With the symptoms of yang deficiency described in this book, you feel tired and cold, even though there is no acute disease.

Some conditions with aspects of yang deficiency as described here include:

- Hypothyroidism

- M.E: myalgic encephalomyelitis: chronic fatigue, though this often contains a syndrome called, in Chinese medicine, 'Damp'

- Some kinds of depression (though not those caused by Qi Stagnation)

- Some forms of obesity

- Many of the effects of diabetes

- Many forms of circulatory disorders

- Some skin disorders, usually those which are worse in the cold

- Dementia (because 'clear' yang energy no longer ascends to the head)

- Heart beat slows – bradycardia – or becomes unreliable, possibly with ectopic beats or palpitations (though palpitations can be due to excess yang unregulated by yin)

- Many age-related conditions: as your vigour reduces you become slower, thinking takes longer, your former decisiveness deteriorates, you cannot defend yourself so well, you become bent and cannot stand upright properly

- Fatigue from overwork: many people experience this from time to time. It often produces a dull headache, tired eyes, scalp sensitivity and a tendency to slump. The headache of this type recovers briefly if you close your eyes, apply pressure to or stroke your head. However, to clear the symptoms, you need rest (sleep) and nourishment, typically in that order

- Parkinson's, as both yin and yang reduce, although here yin reduces more than yang, leading to general weakness but a tremor due to lack of yin (Blood[21] deficiency) more than lack of yang

- Many sleep disorders produce these yang deficiency symptoms as a secondary effect

- Some forms of mental disability, where thinking clearly or logically is difficult, making it hard to articulate thoughts and describe ideas and feelings: what used to be called cretinism probably fits this description.

---

21. http://www.acupuncture-points.org/blood.html

CHAPTER 6

Ageing and Yang Deficiency

When young, your body is small and its yang resources pro-portionately larger than when your body is full-grown. So yang manifests more easily, poorly restrained by yin. Yang is there-fore less well controlled, which you see in the tantrums and restless behaviour of the young.

The young are also more susceptible to yang influences, such as excitement and the sun. Beware exposure too soon to heat and sunlight: babies easily over-heat and burn. (Conversely, healthy babies are more tolerant of cold than their parents, who often swaddle them with too much clothing.)

If teenagers seek a tan, encourage them to keep active while getting it. Take them swimming or walking or encourage them to play sports: the activity uses up some of their excess yang. Just sitting skin-exposed to the sun to roast is a recipe for ill-ness, as many find when they lie in the sun ill-advisedly.

Most people indulge the young in their wilfulness, passions and casual attitude towards consequences. Everyone makes mistakes in their teenage years, and even later: typical of yang. Healthy young flesh is supple and moist, colourful, firm and vibrant, a wonderful mix of yang and yin. When yin is deficient, or yang in excess, you may get exuberance of yang which, depending on our viewpoint can be life-enhancing – as in mad enthusiasm and passion – or destructive, as in vandalism.

Aging depletes both yang and yin.

You notice the **yin** deficiencies in wasting flesh, the drying out of natural fluids, skin and joints, the withering of the body, the reduction in bulk, the loss of healthy roundness and resilience. Memory and attention suffer as the brain loses neural connections. Poor sleep patterns reduce endurance.

At the same time, you notice **yang** deficiency: people slow down, react less quickly, become more dependent on others, and often feel colder. Concentration and imagination are poorer. They tire more quickly and need frequent rests.

It also shows in the reduced ardour, less sexual energy, more cautiousness and 'wisdom' – both are yin words – but these yin states are caused by reduced yang: in other words, the previous balance of yin and yang now appears as more yin, because of yang deficiency.

Because there is less yang, less warmth, the Blood circulates less efficiently, often leading to Blood Stasis[1], which in Chinese medicine is implicated in many conditions of ageing.

This reduction in yang occurs mainly because the body's source of yang depletes as you age. Called your 'jing-essence[2], this is the name in Chinese medicine for what is considered to be your most precious inherited asset.

Some of us are fortunate in having plenty of jing-essence. We use it up fast during acute illness, periods of severe strain, from over-lifting and over-working for too long, when the food we eat is inadequate and we have to survive on our inner resources, during times of acute stress, war and privation, and as we age.

The younger we are when this happens, the faster we recover, although a very severe illness in early youth can be a major impediment to health and energy for many years after, and in some cases, for life.

1. http://www.acupuncture-points.org/blood-stasis.html
2. http://www.acupuncture-points.org/jing-essence.html'

Not so, if we are much older: we do not recover so easily. That means we must take more care in what we do. We must drive and walk more carefully, eat more slowly to extract the nutrients we need, be more sparing in the use of drugs and medications. Why? Because we lack the bounce of yang supported by a resilient yin. Lacking that bounce, our bodies recover more slowly.

Basically, to combat yin deficiency, you need more good nutrition, rest and sleep. These help yin which can then go on to recover yang.

For yang deficiency, you may also need stimulation and change, neither of which, as you age, may you be pleased to receive.

Even so, the most important factor for health is yang. If the spirit is strong, it can handle physical deficiencies. Keeping up the spirits of ageing people is, for carers, their most important function: helping patients approach death with the right outlook for a peaceful transition, and enjoying their later years with a positive outlook that is an inspiration to all.

Some organisations have recognised the need for this, and gradually some government agencies are realising how spiritual health means people are happier as they age, with better health and more ability to surmount the problems of old age. Consequently, and importantly for governments, they are cheaper as regards their health and social needs.

Of course, in the short run, biddable people, ie those with low levels of yang, are easier to handle. They cause less trouble. But the theory of yin and yang suggests that more health resources will be needed for them, as they become ever more dependent.

The longer people can look after themselves the better: they retain their yang faculties more easily if challenged to care for themselves. Once institutionalised, ideally they should still be allowed, so far as possible, to wash, move and feed themselves.

The worst way to care for them is to park them in front of a television!

When older, and becoming both yin and yang deficient, the warmth of the sun is often welcome, but its rays can be damaging to old, yin-deficient bodies. So, as with very young, sun exposure is good but needs to be rationed to avoid sunburn and drying out. Young bodies quickly produce signs of sunburn because they already have lots of yang energy, which the sun easily exacerbates, drying and burning. Old bodies take longer to produce symptoms, so all the more important to monitor their exposure on hot sunny days: their problem is a lack of both yin and yang. They like the warmth of the yang-sun, but their yin-deficient bodies take longer to react to the burning rays and their nerve systems (also yin in quality) are more deficient, so they don't realise in time that they are burning.

Put another way, babies and children have small yin bodies but plenty of yang, so are easily damaged by too much yang. Older people have bodies where their yin has dried out or shrunk: they must also take care against excess yang.

The same applies mentally. Young people are easily over-excited, and then cannot sleep. Telling your small children that tomorrow morning you are taking them to Disneyland will probably stop them from sleeping!

For older people, because their bodies are shrinking (less yin), they are more prone to worry, anxiety and insomnia. So older people suffer based on the same principle. In fact, older people can be both yin deficient (shrinking bodies) and yang deficient, (cold and in low spirits.)

However, we must still nurture what we have, so taking care means not just having regard for yin but also for yang: we should have something in life that excites or enthuses us, something to look forward to, to hope for, someone or something to love. And we should try to foster a welcoming heart that is open to new experiences and forgiving of the past.

Hence, the importance of good spiritual health, a positive attitude, and the sun.

CHAPTER 7

Yin opposes Yang

Yin excess type of Yang Deficiency

Not only physical invasions by cold prevent yang from flourishing: you may be someone who is naturally slow to anger and is reliable and steady in life! There is a fine balance between being like this and being too 'slow', for instance:

- slow thinker, or perhaps someone who thinks for too long before deciding or acting

- lacking enterprise or motivation, happy to 'go with the flow': some might say apathetic or lazy

- ... or just a bit sluggish

- likes eating and takes less exercise than necessary to prevent weight gain

- tends to oversleep

- rather set in your ways: inclined to enjoy ritual and tried and tested habits (even though these may be good ones!)

- prefer the same kind of holiday each year, preferably not doing much except sleeping and eating

Some of these traits may look like hypothyroidism, but your thyroid may be perfectly healthy! You are just like this and for long-term health this is not a bad place to be: you are less likely to die from accidents brought on by impetuosity.

If this is you then you are probably someone with good strong yin reserves – or you may just be growing older, and possibly wiser. If you feel or are led to believe that you should improve yourself by becoming more yang like, the following (mostly physical) activities may help:

- interval training: this makes your heart work hard for short periods of time alternating with slower or resting periods. It can be done in many kinds of sports, including running, 'cardio' exercise machines, cycling, swimming, even walking

- setting goals that stretch you but are satisfying and rewarding – such as giving yourself a time limit to write an article or book, then pushing yourself to complete it within the time set

- learning to dance fast: it hardly matters what kind of dance, except that it requires quick movement

- learning a competitive sport that requires fast physical reactions, such as judo, wrestling, tennis, squash: (gardening and golf are unsuitable!)

- rock-climbing or even mountaineering: requires strength – which you can probably develop – and agility: very rewarding when you reach the top

- joining adventure groups who do things that are out of your comfort zone. They might include sports-training holidays, bungee jumping, wind-surfing, skiing

- learning to play computer games against other people. However, although these may speed up your brain's reflexes, they do little for your cardiovascular system except flood it with adrenaline and cortisol. Neither is beneficial unless you also take exercise to dissipate the hormones!

Full Cold

Reminder: do not confuse yang deficiency with what in Chinese medicine is described as 'full-cold[1]'. As explained before, Full-cold is the name given to a condition where a pathogenic factor has taken over your health, sometimes – but certainly not always – a bacterial or viral infection, making you feel icy-cold.

Usually, this full-cold condition does not improve when warmth is applied, or at least, not for some time, whereas a yang deficient patient likes warmth and usually feels a little better for it immediately. Also, the pain that 'full-cold' produces is intense, much worse than the usual pains from yang deficiency, which are dull.

Full-cold conditions, if they persist, can lead on to yang deficiency.

Other Factors

Extreme cold is dangerous to yang. Ideally it should stimulate us into vigorous action to dispel or avoid it. The most effective defence is a good supply of warmth which means we need to wear plenty, to eat warming foods, and to keep physically active. Warm, encouraging company also helps.

However, although extreme cold is one of the fastest ways to weaken yang, extended periods of exposure even to mild cold can, over time, deplete your yang resources.

If you have poor circulation, other than poor genes it may be that you wore too little at some time in your life, or you wore yourself out through frequent overwork, lack of sleep, or overstrain.

1. http://www.acupuncture-points.org/cold.html

Saturated fats contain yang energy that your body needs to remain warm and active. Unsaturated fats, also important, are the forms of fat we are most often encouraged to eat, but humans have eaten saturated fats for hundreds of thousands of years and still need them.

Saturated fats come from animal fats, including cheese and butter, coconut oils and nuts; also from some fatty vegetables like avocado, (which also contains unsaturated fats).

(Do not eat what are called trans-fats, also called hydro-genated vegetable fats. These are industrially produced fats with extra hydrogen forced into them to make them solid at room temperature when normally they would be liquid. This makes them easy to store, inexpensive to produce, durable for long periods and highly profitable for manufacturers. They are poisonous, whatever manufacturers have said in the past to the contrary.)

Damp

When yang is deficient, many other bodily and state functions begin to fail.

In the body, for instance, Spleen Yang fails to 'transform' food, or is overwhelmed by cold, wet conditions. This leads to what is called 'Damp[2]'. There is heaviness, soreness and swelling: many forms of arthritis share these symptoms, for example. At the same time, digestion is weakened and energy depleted. Eventually the Spirit, yang, is diminished.

Other Factors that weaken Yang

Many factors can weaken yang, including:

• Slow insidious diseases and conditions

2. http://www.acupuncture-points.org/damp.html

- Streptococcus or staphylococcus infections that produce focal infections or invade connective tissues like tendons and valves causing sprains and prolapses
- Drug and alcohol abuse
- Over-use of stimulants, including coffee (for more on coffee see under Bitter flavour in the section on Nutrition in Chapter 8)
- Frequent or prolonged use of antibiotics or other medication
- Long periods of depression and anxiety or stress
- Too many dairy products
- Too many foods containing the sweet flavour, including sugar
- Chemotherapy
- Radiation therapy (In Chinese medicine, radiation is heating, so is drying: this depletes yin resources, which therefore cannot support yang)
- Immune-suppressant medication

Fear

Terror and extreme fear can make us defecate and urinate involuntarily. Yang energy, which should hold these effluents in place, is pushed downwards by strong fear, and bodily wastes just 'fall out'. This makes us shake and quiver: our clear yang energy, which should rise to our heads and keep our brains clear, is dragged away and down.

Consequently, we cannot think straight, our bodies are uncontrollable and/or our heart races, stops and starts: signs of yin being unable to regulate, adjust or repair scattered yang.

This 'scattered' yang needs rest and reassurance, sometimes treatment, to assist recovery.

Trauma

Accidents disturb our spirit and scatter our energy. In Chinese medicine, they cause what is called Blood Stasis[3], which we observe as bruises, though in Chinese medicine the concept behind the words 'Blood stasis' goes much deeper than that.

Our yang energy's main job is to defend us. When an accident happens, our yang energy can become fragmented. How fast we recover depends on our yin reserves, the quality and balance of our yin and yang, time, rest and our spirit.

Violence done to you in youth, whether mental or physical, may have long-term consequences.

With 'scattered' yang and Blood Stasis, you can go to pieces very easily.

In Western medical understanding, this category would include any kind of shock or trauma causing adrenal gland exhaustion.

I have seen patients who suffered huge damage earlier in their lives. But for treatment, the pattern of their personality disturbance and physical pain would have continued indefinitely. Very often they lacked confidence, and their posture, appearance and behaviour were altered detrimentally.

If you have suffered trauma, think carefully about how your health, energy and life changed after it. The symptoms associated with Blood Stasis can take time to appear, so sometimes you must look back over a period of months or even years to notice changes. These are far more than the disappearance of bruising or scars. They can affect your whole character.

What to do about it? Mending Blood Stasis takes time, even with good treatment. Then comes the process of encouraging the spirit to realise it is free.

In Chinese medicine, for health after trauma

- the Blood must be able to move properly again,

3. http://www.acupuncture-points.org/blood-stasis.html

- the channels of acupuncture need to be 'cleared' to let the Qi flow along them smoothly

- the Zangfu (ie organ energies) must be rebalanced to provide both mental and physical energy

- The Spirit must be encouraged to manifest again

- Nowadays there are also psychological ways to do this, but time spent with congenial and supportive friends or family also works for many

- Quiet meditation and prayer suits some

- I have known the right homoeopathic remedy transform a life

- The various methods of treatment available to practitioners of Asian medicine can be hugely beneficial

- Learning how to feed, rest, exercise and hold the body (ie posture) provides the yin vessel for the yang spirit to flourish

- Tai Chi and Yoga may help you, over time, by taking you gently to your limits

Over-strain

The kind of overstrain that mainly causes yang deficiency is that of physical over-strain, eg over-lifting, especially if unfit or too young. However, physical over-strain covers a multiple of sins:

- Training too hard for a sport without taking proper breaks and rests to let your body recover. Many body-builders and runners wonder why, despite a frenzy of nutritional supplements, they always feel exhausted. They should take more days off between training sessions to allow their bodies to recuperate.

- Over-partying usually means staying up late night after night.

Fun at the time but the result is a lack of sleep and yang deficiency. (Of course, drugs are often taken to intensify and prolong the party spirit, leading to still greater exhaustion.)

- One need not be a body-builder or party-goer to over-strain oneself. The very occasional football game or tug of war can deplete yang because the body is not trained for it and the effort is too great.

The same goes for people who don't actually over-lift but do a variety of activities every day, racing from one thing to the next, never stopping to rest. Each activity requires intense concentration, like a search-light. Mental overwork exhausts yin more than yang, but this kind of mental work, rushing from one thing to the next, also exhausts yang as much as, or more than, yin. (I found that I lost yang energy more than yin energy when I was seeing patients, each for short periods, one after the next for many hours on end, day after day. In most cases I was sitting talking and listening to the patients who came for treatment. Each required my intense concentration and intellectual effort, but none of them for long. As I say, this seemed to deplete my yang energy more than my yin energy. I could keep doing it for weeks, but I lost my bounce and, with hindsight, became a bit depressed.)

Disappointment, Criticism

- Yang energy is deflated and reduced by adverse factors like disappointment and criticism.
- Your enthusiasms are not shared by others
- Your enterprise and initiative are viewed with indifference or criticism
- Your passion is not returned

- Your self-confidence is put down by powerful adverse forces
- Your youthful fun is met with boredom and apathy
- Your hopes are dashed
- Your intuitions turn out to be wrong

We have all had this happen to us! How you react depends on your resources, on your family and background and on your sense of identity.

CHAPTER 8

Yin supports Yang: Nutrition

How to Reduce Yang Deficiency

In chapter 2 you read about the 'rules' for yin and yang.
    The first rule, see Chapter 7, is when Yin *opposes* Yang.
    This chapter is about Rule 2: Yin *supports* Yang.

Rest

To yang deficient people lack of rest is not an obvious cause of their problem. Rest and sleep are boring. In fact, this cause of yang deficiency is actually a consequence of yin deficiency.

Some athletes and sports-people may wonder why they always have minor health issues such as allergies or food sensitivities, runny noses, post-nasal phlegm and mild headaches. These are often the result of yang stimulating activities that exhaust yin.

Because they are apparently so fit and have such strong determination and self-discipline they ignore these minor health problems. They continue to train, often blaming poor nutrition or health allergies.

Often these are not really nutritional or allergy problems: they are just pushing themselves beyond their natural limits.

To be a great athlete requires you to push your limits, but the result can be that your yang energy, the kind of energy that also manifests in the immune force, becomes too weak to keep health problems at bay.

These minor health problems show that the athlete's body is near its limit. This means that it may take only a small extra stimulus, such as a shock or an accident (to which in this state they will be more prone), to put them out of action.

How much sleep is adequate? People vary, of course, but if you are very yang deficient, you probably need at least 8 hours nightly, of which at least a third is deep sleep.

If your sleep is poor[1], you may find that Chinese medicine helps to explain it.

Training and Practice

How we are brought up makes a huge difference to our ability to balance yin and yang.

Having a loving family behind us is the first requirement but how we are taught and trained can compensate for many deficiencies. If trained to channel our yang energies creatively we become stronger and less inclined to waste or dissipate them.

Training implies repetition and practice. The armed forces are huge yin resources with a yang function. They take in the young, and discipline this source of yang so that it can be used effectively in battle. Instead of the young wasting their energies in youthful folly(!), they learn to survive in perilous situations and to work together in combat.

Used this way, they become a deadly fighting force: applied yang.

If you take a bit of iron, with knowledge and resources, using

1. http://www.acupuncture-points.org/insomnia.html

the right stones you may sharpen it to a fine edge and point. Now, that lump of iron has become a lethal weapon.

Proper training and practice instil discipline that husbands yang. Training should include how

- to breathe properly and fully, in both chest and abdomen
- to stand or sit with good posture
- to strengthen the body, especially the upper body and back

These take work but immediately incline the body and mind towards better yang energy.

Ritual

Rites and rituals are hugely important ways we order our lives. In religious settings they are the physical expression of a perceived higher order.

We teach rituals to children, for example:

- How to brush teeth
- Manners expected when eating
- How to worship, meditate or pray
- When to sleep
- How to order the day, via meals, school/work, exercise, play and sleep
- The rules of games
- Good practice when driving cars
- How to behave in assemblies, classes, congregations, crowds, queues

They are signs of civilisation. They are accepted modes of

behaviour, so yin. Young people often resent them. Older people value them.

As people retire and become more sedate in their lives, attending a regular religious service may at first be merely a need for company. However, for some, the spiritual side can become more meaningful, leading to a more peaceable and contented life. Here the yang energy balances the yin body as it becomes smaller and more frail. The ritual helps them assimilate the spiritual side.

According to one of Chinese medicines most ancient theories, the 'Four phase' or 'Five Element' theory, these rituals and their potential for spiritual strength come under the Metal element, that of the Lungs and Large Intestine, the organ energies that are connected with the absorption of Qi and the ability to discard what is not needed, the latter itself becoming the matter for future life. See also chapter 18.

NUTRITION AND YANG DEFICIENCY

In Chinese medicine, foods, like herbs, are described in various ways. The two main such ways are according to a food's effect on the warmth of the body, i.e the food's energy, such as warming or cooling, and according to its 'flavour' (bitter, sweet, pungent, salty, sour).

For health, take both into account.

While the food's energy has a more short-term effect on the body; its flavour provides the ancient equivalent of nutrition. For someone yang deficient even the most nutritious food will not help much if the food has a very cold energy, because he lacks enough yang energy to digest it. Equally, if he ate only warm-type foods of one flavour or category, his health would not improve and might get worse – just as someone who eats only 'sweet' foods will eventually get sick.

Usually, when strengthening Yang it is better first to reduce the number of cooling, moistening foods (yin qualities) than to increase or emphasise warming, drying foods (yang qualities). (This is a consequence of Rule 1 of the four rules set out in chapter 2.)

In any case, the body is both yin and yang, and needs a range of foods to flourish. But yang deficient people should reduce or avoid 'cold' foods and eat an otherwise balanced diet.

Why? If there is yang deficiency, the yin energy has been unable to replenish it, so the yin energy needs support too, which comes from the balanced diet. Perhaps one could say that your yang energy levels have more to do with the food energy (hot or cold) and your yin energy comes more from with the balance of your diet.

A small reminder for those who skipped reading this book up to here ...

Although this book has a number of suggestions, the single most important and effective way to recover yang is to get adequate rest and sleep – see earlier in this chapter.

Food

But good food is also essential, and the time, ability and circumstances to digest it. All the yang food in the world will be wasted if it goes straight through you, as it may if your body is unable to absorb and exploit the nutrients it provides.

For example, very spicy or hot food (yang qualities in food) may be hard to digest and lead to diarrhoea, with only a temporary heating reaction. This is temporary because it makes you perspire: that cools you, in time depleting both your yin and yang energies.

Some foods/herbs are thought to increase libido. In some people they do, in others not. Putting aside the placebo effect, it would be strange if every such food was always effective for everyone. We are all different and our bodies – and minds – respond to different things.

In fact, our bodies change from day to day. The whole circumstances have to be taken into account. Fortunes are spent to increase libido, which is a product of a healthy balance between yin and yang[2], Blood[3] and Qi[4] backed by strong jing-essence[5] and with all the different zangfu[6] organs working properly and in balance.

(Why *all* of the zang-fu organs? Surely some are more important for libido than others? Yes, but although less important in this situation than the Heart[7] and Liver[8], the Large Intestine and its associated acupuncture channels can still ruin the day if your skin is bad, you have a headache and are constipated!)

Food Energy

The main foods to reduce are cold, iced and chilled foods/drinks: especially in winter or in cold conditions. Also reduce raw foods, such as salads and raw fruit. Raw foods have great qualities and normally, in health, are good foods. But when you are yang deficient, being cold, these foods are harder to digest. Replace those salads and raw fruits with cooked vegetables, eaten warm.

If you cannot avoid them, drink some warm liquids before eating the cold foods. For instance, take some warm tea, or hot soup, beforehand. These increase the Yang available to your Stomach and Spleen, reducing the cooling effect of the foods that follow. Finish the meal with more warm liquid.

2. http://www.acupuncture-points.org/yin-and-yang.html
3. http://www.acupuncture-points.org/blood.html
4. http://www.acupuncture-points.org/qi.html
5. http://www.acupuncture-points.org/jing-essence.html
6. http://www.acupuncture-points.org/zang-fu.html
7. http://www.acupuncture-points.org/heart.html
8. http://www.acupuncture-points.org/liver-functions.html

If you are yang deficient, do not drink water, especially if it is cold, chilled or iced, when eating meals. It reduces the little amount of Stomach yang that you have. Drink water between meals, but drink it warm, not chilled.

How a food is prepared and cooked makes a huge difference. Cooking, generally speaking, increases yang. Roasting and frying are even more yang. Adding liquid or cooling and freezing a food makes it more yin in action.

Yang energy is reduced by eating too much food at a time, even if not cold: you feel lethargic and ill or bloated, or get bowel disturbances such as loose stools that contain undigested matter. This effect would be worse if you were tired when you ate.

Of course, on a hot day, even in winter, someone with mild yang deficiency can usually manage some cold or chilled food without getting ill. But it is easy to make a mistake and take too much! When you are yang deficient and hungry, your body inclines you to eat more, even if the food's energy is wrong for you. An imbalanced body energy/health is easily further imbalanced (just as when you stand on one leg, I can easily push you over.)

As already explained, yang deficient people should avoid cool, chilled or frozen food, especially on cold days. They should eat cooked food, and they should eat it warm. They should always chew it all carefully before swallowing. Chewing and the action of stomach acids is yang in nature: they break down the food into smaller parts that are easier to digest.

TO OBTAIN MORE YANG, CHEW!

As the yang deficiency improves, the body will cope better with cold-type foods and foods eaten raw, cold or chilled.

If yang deficient, it is, however, a mistake to eat only foods with yang quality because all good foods contain nutrition that the body needs. To make yang the body draws on both yin and yang foods. A car needs coolants (yin) and oil (comparatively yin) as well as fuel (yang). If you use no coolant or oil your car will soon break down.

Even traditional Chinese herbal formulae intended mainly to assist yang contain herbs that also nourish and protect yin.

Reminder! Just as a bucket of water will extinguish a candle, so will a large meal, or eating too fast, either test or weaken your yang energy. When yang deficient, never eat a huge meal, and certainly not when tired. If you are tired and hungry, eat a snack first (for example a handful of nuts or an oatcake with butter or even cheese – but not too much!). Then wait a while.

This was probably the original purpose of appetisers or the first course of a meal, usually smaller than the rest. They should be small enough to be easily and quickly digested to give you enough energy to digest the main dishes when they appear.

Then, in theory – a bit later, when it comes to the meal itself, your body will have picked up enough energy to digest it. But even here, do not eat a huge meal if the hour is late. In the evenings, unless you are on holiday or well-rested, large meals put a strain on your system's yang energy. Large meals are better eaten earlier, before you get tired.

Of course, modern chefs now show off so that the first course may not always work as originally intended. Also, nowadays the appetiser is often sour or even bitter, to stimulate hunger.

Food Flavours

In Chinese and other East Asian forms of medicine (most of which rely on Chinese medicine or the ancient texts it is based on) there are five basic flavours or tastes: bitter, sweet, pungent or acrid, salty, sour. All foods are classified as belonging to one or more of these tastes.

For health, one should regularly eat a range of foods representing each of the tastes, preferably grown naturally – organically, because the ancient Chinese lacked modern artificial fertilisers, let alone herbicides and fungicides etc. The foods they used were grown or harvested from natural, often wild, sources.

Eating foods from all groups leads to balance between the different organ energies – the zang-fu – which, being in balance, will incline you less to binge-eat.

If you are yang deficient, of these flavours you will almost certainly be drawn towards the sweet, pungent and possibly salty tastes and the foods classified as such. These belong, respectively to the Earth, Metal and Water phases, about which more is written in chapter 18 from a different perspective.

Not all benefit yang.

By the way, in the following you will notice some foods appearing in several places. Apple, for example, is classified as both sour and sweet-tasting. If you eat a variety of apples you will already know this from experience!

For more on individual foods, see the Appendix for tables.

Sweet flavoured foods

Sweet tasting food gives you a quick lift!

As babies, we encounter this taste first in our mother's milk. The sweet taste is programmed into our systems as relating to nourishment.

But now we have too much of it, sugar being so widely available. Eating too much sweet food, especially containing added sugar, produces metabolic changes which can lead to diabetes, obesity and a range of more serious conditions.

Nevertheless, we definitely do need sweet tasting foods as so classified in Chinese medicine, but not foods made sweet by the addition of sweeteners, including sugar, or sweetened by prolonged cooking, as with fruit.

Sweet-tasting foods, according to Chinese medicine, include:
abalone
apple
carp fish
carrot
cherry
chestnut
corn
dates
glutinous rice
grapes
Honey
longan aril
lotus seed
milk
peanut
pears
peas
potato
pumpkin
rice
shiitake mushroom
soybean
sugar cane
sweet potato
taro
wheat

These sweet foods fall into two broad categories:

1/ Nourishing, but neutral or warm in temperature. These include:

- legumes (for example peas and beans)

- meat (in China these were traditionally mainly chicken and pork)
- nuts
- starchy vegetables

These are mostly beneficial for yang deficient people.
2/ Mostly neutral or cooling, which includes

- dairy foods
- most fruit
- sugar, honey and other sweeteners: these have a steadying, calming effect – hence their use to calm children of all ages. Overuse means the metabolism has to speed up to use the extra energy, provoking hyperactivity of many kinds, none of them beneficial to a resilient quality in yang, followed by quick depression, now recognised as due to excess insulin as the body strives to maintain its blood sugar concentration within normal levels.
- potatoes
- rice and most other grains

These are less beneficial for yang deficient people, and too much may be harmful.

Too Much Sweet-flavoured food?

In general, too much of the sweet taste is said to injure the muscles. In some people this can mean loss of weight, but more commonly in developed countries where there are bountiful amounts of sweet food it causes additional flesh lacking muscles or muscular tone, and more fat.

Many sports people depend on high quantities of 'sweet

flavour' food for energy and muscular growth. When they stop performing, or grow older and less able to metabolise it, their muscles deteriorate unless they reduce the quantity of foods of this sweet flavour.

Salty Tasting Food

Salty foods are said to be cooling and they help your body regulate its fluid levels for health. You need some salt-flavour food in your diet, but as a yin energy food, too much of it is not beneficial if you are yang deficient.

Too much salty-flavoured food is said to injure the Blood: in terms of Western medicine this comes close to the adverse effect too much salt has on circulation and the heart organ.

Salty flavour foods include:

Abalone
amaranths
barley
crabs
cuttlefish
dried mussel
duck meat
ham
jellyfish, preserved
kelp
laver
millet
oyster
pigeon's egg
pig's blood
pig's bone marrow
pig's organs
pork
razor clam

sea clams
sea cucumber
sea shrimps
seaweed
snail
Soya sauce

Pungent or acrid flavour foods

You might think that pungent foods, which help your body push energy up and out, often by making you perspire, would be good for yang deficient people. Indeed, pungent food often does help them feel better for a while, but the cooling effect of perspiration, even though they don't notice it much, is less beneficial.

In Chinese medicine, pungent tasting foods are often used to help the body increase its metabolic rate to fight off bacteria and bugs. For example, pungent herbs are used in herbal formulae to combat a syndrome known as invasion of Wind-Cold[9], recognised in Chinese medicine since antiquity: when you read its symptoms you will realise that Wind-Cold is very much with us today.

Pungent flavoured foods include:
Cabbage (Shanghai)
Celery
Chili pepper
Chives (Chinese)
Cinnamon
Coriander
Curry
Fennel
Garlic
Ginger (fresh)

9. http://www.acupuncture-points.org/wind-cold.html

Kumquat
Leeks
Mustard leaves and seeds
Onion
Pepper (cayenne)
Peppercorn (Sichuan-type)
Radish leaf
Spearmint
Tangerine peel
Taro
Turnip
Wine

These foods move qi and circulate blood. They disperse mucus from the lungs. These are yang qualities, but on their own, or if over-eaten, they do not lead to a lasting increase in yang in the body. In fact, taking too much acrid or pungent-tasting food is known to 'injure' your Qi, meaning you have less energy.

So by all means eat more of these foods if you are yang-deficient, but not too many of the most strongly pungent ones listed.

However, if you are yang deficient, a safe herb to add to your diet is raw ginger. This, added in small quantities regularly to what you eat, helps your Spleen and Stomach energies turn what you eat into what you need. Compared to coffee (see below), it works more slowly but its action does not lead, as with coffee, to yin deficiency when taken in normal doses.

As mentioned, very spicy foods, such as chillies and peppers, also benefit yang. But they can easily become too heating, making you perspire and thereby cooling you, the opposite of what you need for a steady improvement in yang. The same goes for hot curries. If they don't make you perspire, they may hasten the movement of food through your intestines, leading to explosive diarrhoea or more frequent urgings to move your bowels.

The Sour Taste

Adjust your diet to include more of the foods and tastes represented by the Wood and Fire phases, these being yang phases. Respectively, these are foods of the sour and bitter taste. You do not need much of them, but by including them in your diet you will eventually find you have less desire for the sweet, pungent and salty flavoured foods.

apple
grapes
hawthorn fruit
lemon
loquat fruit
mango
olives
oranges
papaya
peaches
pears
pineapple
plums
pomegranate
pomelo
royal jelly
sauerkraut
strawberry
tangerines
tomatoes
vinegar

If you have understood me so far, you may find the list above confusing, because most of the foods listed are fruits, which, at least when eaten raw the normal way, are cooling. Well, yes! But as explained, we are talking here about the food quality, not its energy, and you need comparatively few of them. Several of them can be taken warm, such as sauerkraut and vinegar.

Also, do realise that the more imbalanced your health is, the less choice you have.

Cider vinegar

Of sour tasting foods, the prime example is apple cider vinegar, preferably organic and unfiltered, because filtering removes some of its most beneficial qualities. Take some of this daily. It has a gently tonifying effect on your digestion and helps to clear your head, meaning it enables your body to send more yang energy upwards and clear poor energy downwards. It is easy to take and widely available. You only need a couple of dessert-spoons of it daily in warm water to notice benefit.

Sour tasting foods stimulate your gall-bladder and liver to work more efficiently. Strong Gallbladder[10] energy is associated in Chinese medicine with courage, quick reactions, effective and objective discrimination, good sight and foresight. The Gallbladder is also related to healthy tendons, giving physical confidence and resilience to trauma. These are yang qualities.

Fermented food

Another excellent representative of the sour taste is fermented food, such as sauerkraut. Fermenting was traditionally used in many countries to preserve food, but it was slow: after cleaning, shredding and pickling your cabbage in brine, you sealed it in a hole in the ground to maintain a steady, low temperature.

Then you waited a few months while the bacteria and yeasts fought it out, at which point, if the seal was still unbroken,

10. http://www.acupuncture-points.org/gallbladder-deficiency.html

the resultant sauerkraut was highly nutritious. Fermented food contains enzymes to help you digest it, it has many good pro- biotics, it contains vitamin C, and it has a very long shelf life.

Small amounts of fermented food help tone the digestion, helping to clear excess acidity and introducing a huge range of beneficial organisms that improve health.

These organisms help your immune system defend you bet- ter: an important yang function.

Bitter Tasting Foods

As mentioned, we have grown accustomed to foods in the sweet and salty spectrum. Increasingly we like pungent foods and some sour foods too, but we eat few bitter-tasting foods, perhaps because bitterness is associated with poison. However, for health we do need some bitter-tasting foods. The bitter taste is said, in Chinese medicine, to drain heat, dry dampness and descend qi.

What that means is that where there is excess heat in the body, either from extreme exertion or appearing as inflamma- tion, foods with a bitter taste will help the body cope with it.

Bitter-tasting foods also help the body to clear damp, rep- resented by feelings of heaviness, often with swelling, such as when there is poor circulation. This highlights the relationship between the bitter taste and the Heart. Tea's bitter taste is milder than that of coffee, but both stimulate the Heart to cir- culate blood.

Descending Qi has several meanings but the most recogniz- able is the ability to induce bowel movements.

Unfortunately, bitter-tasting foods are not abundant. The list below shows that for most of us, it is various kinds of cabbage and celery that are the easiest to find. Many people dislike these vegetables.

The following lists some foods with the 'bitter' taste.

almonds, bitter
apricot seed
arrowhead
asparagus
bergamot
bitter gourd
cabbage – various kinds including brussel sprouts
dark chocolate
celery leaves
coffee
dandelion leaf
gingko
Indian lettuce
lily bulb
lotus leaf
peach kernel
pig's liver
plum kernel
seaweed
tea leaf
turnips
vinegar
wild cucumber
Wine

We have one abundant and strong source of the bitter taste, commonly used. In the absence of foods many of us dislike, we substitute coffee, often in excessive quantities.

Coffee is to the Bitter taste as refined white sugar is to the Sweet taste. It is a purified version, lacking the nutritive qualities of real food. By taking too much of it, we over-stimulate yang because there is no yin benefit from it. This short-term benefit has long-term deleterious consequences, which in Chinese medicine may lead to yin deficiency. Eventually this weakens yang as well. Then you have deficiency of both yin and of yang!

For more on the theory behind long-term consequences of repeated quantities of a herb or food, read up on the primary and secondary effects of food[11].

Overall, unrefined bitter foods help the Heart to function better: very important for your yang energy.

Here's a brief comparison of the stronger forms of the bitter taste.

Caffeine and coffee. Very yang in nature, and tends to drain yin quickly in susceptible people. See below.

Strong chocolate, eg dark chocolate. Some health experts recommend taking a square or more of dark chocolate daily, 'to stimulate and benefit the heart'. A small amount can help to foster yang. Even here, however, too much – for you – may produce signs of yin deficiency, such as a sense of pressure in your head, noises in your ears and insomnia, if you have some yin deficiency already, because your yin energy cannot restrain your body's yang reaction to the dark chocolate.

Ginseng. There are various kinds of ginseng. Renshen: Chinese ginseng, is nearly always combined with other herbs in Chinese herbal prescriptions because it stimulates qi and yang more than yin, and other herbs in the prescription work to balance this. Xi yang shen: 'American' ginseng, also benefits qi, but benefits yin fluids too so is more balanced. (Even so, American ginseng is better combined with other herbs or foods.) Unless you know exactly what your needs are, if yang deficient take American rather than Chinese Ginseng. There will then be less chance of inadvertently further unbalancing your health.

Guarana: this contains much more caffeine than coffee, almost four times as much. As such it is like taking several double expresso coffees on an empty stomach. This is too extreme for most people's balanced health. If you must take guarana, do so only very occasionally.

Of course, there are also social drugs which greatly increase

11. http://www.acupuncture-points.org/primary-and-secondary-actions.html

yang temporarily. These are often hardly, if at all, tolerated legally because they can lead to (self-)destructive behaviour and illness. Many of them are bitter.

By the way! Caffeine is in many painkillers and mood-enhancing concoctions, also in some sports supplements.

If you are in the habit of taking too much caffeine, as in many coffees or colas daily, then probably you are already a bit yang deficient, whether or not you are also yin deficient. And if you also take your caffeine with sugar or artificial sweeteners, then you will also be damaging your Spleen[12] energy.

Probably your best course of action is to stop all caffeine, and go cold-turkey for a few days. If you feel no ill-effects, no tiredness, headache, irritability or sleep difficulties, then congratulate yourself, you were probably not yang deficient! But even so, take less in future. As you age, your constitution weakens and becomes more susceptible to deficiency of both yin and yang, which caffeine easily exacerbates.

Yang Foods

To increase yang energy, after avoiding 'bad' and raw, cold or chilled foods, the single most effective way of increasing both yin and yang is, to repeat myself, to chew your food properly.

The other main consideration if you are yang deficient is to eat food that has been cooked and is warm when eaten.

Below is a table covering many foods, with their qualities in terms of being cold, cooling, neutral, warming or hot. If you are yang deficient, avoid cold foods, and eat mainly those listed as cooling, neutral or warming. Avoid hot foods or take them only in small quantities.

If you eat a food described as cold, eat it when it has been cooked and is still hot.

12. http://www.acupuncture-points.org/spleen.html

For those in a hurry, the following is a rough summary of effects. For more detail on individual foods, see the Appendix.

- Beans: most are neutral, some cooling. Cook well.

- Dairy products (rather frowned upon in Chinese medicine): neutral, some cooling

- Fish: most fish is neutral, some are warming and a few are cold

- Fruit: neutral or cooling (cherries are deemed warming). Fruit is more cooling than most vegetables and because it is mostly eaten raw, it is harder to digest. Bear in mind that fruit is mostly picked in late summer when the weather is still warm, so is an appropriate food then.

- Grains: most are neutral, a few warming, like oats. Cook well. Wheat is not particularly liked in Chinese medicine.

- Herbs, dried: warming. Yang-enhancing herbs include astragalus and oryza seed, cordyceps, walnut, cynamorium songaricum, and ginseng about which see more under bitter foods.

- Meat: most meats are warming or hot, some neutral

- Nuts and seeds: most neutral, some warming. Chew well. Nuts and seeds carry their genetic code for growth and when sprouted, you get them at the earliest stages of growth, a very yang moment in a plant's life. But a little can go a long way. Nuts and seeds are concentrated foods, rather like health supplements!

- Oils and fats: vary. Olive oil and butter are neutral or cooling; walnut oil is warming; safflower and sunflower oils are cooling, soybean oil is warming. Bone marrow oil is warming. Ghee is either neutral or slightly warming. Animal fats[13] like dripping, lard and tallow are warming and very nourishing.

13. http://www.marksdailyapple.com/yet-another-primal-primer-animal-fats

- Salads: cooling

- Spices: warming or hot

- Tea (Indian or Chinese) is cooling. Herb teas, like fennel, tend to be warming.

- Sweeteners (excluding artificial sweeteners, which are not good food and which some think are very bad): mostly neutral or cooling, although too many can be briefly warming. Use sparingly, because too many sweet foods can damage your Spleen energy, on which your body relies heavily to absorb nutrients from what you eat.

- Vegetables: most cooling, a few warming. Cooking them and eating them warm makes them more warming, more yang.

From the above you can see that salads should be eaten only on hot days or when you are feeling very well.

Vegetables and some meats, with added spices or herbs, should suit you well, as do beans, all if well-cooked. Grains are mostly good, but not in large quantities, although admittedly the Chinese eat a lot of rice, it being easy to digest, unlike wheat.

Eat a range of nuts and seeds, chewed well.

Cooking increases the yang qualities of food.

Reduce dairy foods which tend to be a heavy load on your digestion.

From the above, and to summarise, if you are yang deficient, you will realise that Chinese medicine emphasises that you take food that is not too cold, is eaten warm, has been cooked well, and is easy to digest. All foods should be chewed well.

Once again! The single most yang enhancing food? Is not a food: CHEW PROPERLY!

For a longer list, see the tables below.

Foods to Avoid

Junk foods, refined foods, sweet or rich foods. Like refined cereals for breakfast, they give you a quick yang benefit, but this soon burns out, making you eat or snack more. There is no lasting benefit.

Yin Foods to Avoid

If eating foods described in the food energetic tables as cold or cool, either eat less of them, warm them before eating them, or eat other warming foods at the same time. But do not completely avoid them: even cold-type foods have qualities you need.

However, in winter or cold weather, or if you are tired or cold, avoid them.

Herbs

No Western herbs[14] have yet been specifically classified as yang enhancing, but those that are stimulants or circulatory stimulants are warm, penetrating and stimulating, and often have a pungent taste and a dispersing 'movement'. In effect they appear to be yang enhancing.

They include labiates, and parts from tropical plants such as sassafras, cinnamon, camphor and cayenne. Herbs which appear to have a more systemic tonifying effect include Hyssop and Bayberry bark. See a qualified herbalist for the correct prescription covering the different aspects of your conditiob. Although 'natural', herbs used in concentration are *medicines*. Treat them with respect!

14. For more, see 'The Energetics of Western Herbs' by Peter Holmes, published by Artemis, Boulder

Nutrition Summary   If yang deficient:

- eat food and drinks that are cooked and warm when eaten
- avoid cold, chilled or frozen foods or drinks
- keep meal sizes small, especially in the evening
- do not eat large meals when tired
- Chew well

For more on the energy qualities of different foods, see the Appendix.

CHAPTER 9

Using Yang to Support Yang

Food for the Soul

Arguably an even stronger yang energy than the sun is the spirit – that part of ourselves that aspires. Maintaining oneself in good spirits is the single most important thing for happiness and health. This comes down to having a comfortable sense of identity.

For some, belief in a greater Being is vital. For others, having an aim in life and a shared belief system is enough. Many get their yang inspiration from young people or from working in voluntary or charitable endeavours.

Stimulus from another yang or yin source

Another Yang force may, like an external Yin force, stimulate us into becoming more yang, in defence or defiance.

A famous Ju-Jitsu teacher was asked[1] why he was so success-ful. He said that the trick was to identify which kind of person a student was. Basically there were two types, the rubber ball and the seedling.

1. A story told during a talk to the Buddhist Society by Trevor Leggett, a renowned Judo teacher himself, and for 24 years head of the BBC's Japanese division.

- With the rubber ball, the harder you hit it the higher it bounced.
- With the seedling, it needed constant support and encouragement until one day it was a huge tree, impossible to knock over.

Reflecting on this suggests that timing is vital.

An opponent would try to invade and take you over before your defences were in place: this might happen before you were old enough to have your protection or immune system in place, before you had learned to resist attack. At this stage, like a child, you would expect that the equivalent of adult forces would guard you. At this stage also, for most people, support and encouragement would be more appropriate.

Later, as you grew in strength – and the same goes for countries, see Part 2 – testing, training and opposition would become more appropriate. Nobody becomes an Olympian without learning to cope with opposition.

Immunisation?

The case in favour of immunisation is huge. However, doing it before a child's immune system is in place may lead to unforeseen consequences, not least damage to the immune system which, in Chinese medicine, is largely 'governed' by the Lungs[2]. The Lungs also 'govern' respiration, energy, the skin, our voice, and our capacity for enthusiasm (among other things): all part of our identity. These areas may be compromised, I would argue, by inappropriate immunisation procedures, especially if done too early.

2. http://www.acupuncture-points.org/lung-qi.html

Passion

Another aspect of yang deficiency is lack of passion. This may appear as lack of

- physical passion including sexual passion and desire
- alertness and mental reactivity
- mental passion for an idea or cause
- intellectual vigour
- warmth of personality and sunniness of disposition
- playfulness
- imagination

In Chinese medicine, treatment for lack of passion often requires treatment of the so-called Fire channels (Heart, Small Intestine, Pericardium and Three Heater). Treatment includes warmth (in the form of moxibustion[3]) but rest and nourishment are also vital, with a gradual balancing between the different bodily energies, known as the zang-fu[4].

Creativity

To promote yang in our lives, we should find something that inspires us and/or that forces us to change.

- Artistic creativity is available to nearly everyone, no matter how poor our talents. The result does not have to be good enough for others to hear, view or buy – just creating it may give us pleasure and help us to think differently. For example, painting and shaping, as in pottery and sculpture.

3. http://www.acupuncture-points.org/moxibustion.html
4. http://www.acupuncture-points.org/zang-fu.html

- Music: playing an instrument helps balance our thinking processes and assists yang release in our lives
- Gardening can be creative too – even keeping plants in a pot: consider the Japanese art of Niwaki, of tree-shaping, for example. However, the physical side of gardening is not particularly yang, requiring strength rather than speed.
- Writing or telling stories, perhaps to the young
- Cooking: exploring new tastes and textures, foreign cuisines and foods, can be immensely creative and satisfying
- Photography
- Setting up a small business, a side-line to your main occupation
- Volunteering to help others or a cause
- Enrolling in a course to learn something new for you, from philosophy to geology
- Learning a new language
- Joining a group to discuss books you have read, or dreams you have experienced, or projects to benefit your community

Ideally your activity should make you passionate enough to want to tell others, to inspire them too. If you become an authority on the subject, however, you may find yourself becoming more yin-like in your pronouncements. It is better to remain childlike, even a little innocent!

More adventurously,

- You could try learning to do things a completely different way, such as writing with the other hand.
- Or learn to move your feet anti-clockwise while moving your hands clockwise, and then each independently of the others!

- If you do marathons, take up orienteering ... If you do orienteering, take up ... !

In other words, explore and diversify your talents. The point is that the most yang part of you, your brain and its thought processes, leads your body. If your brain enjoys life, your body will start to do so too.

As a brain surgeon said to one of his musical patients, 'keep playing the organ, it's candy for your brain!'

Activity

Yin is basically inert without yang to warm and move it.

Keeping active means both physically and mentally active. Ideally start young, not suddenly when old, but starting at any age is better than nothing.

Physically, activity should stretch but not strain us. This is why Tai Chi is so beneficial: it keeps us moving and on our feet, it makes us bend and stretch up to but not beyond our boundaries and there is a huge psychological benefit as well.

Above all, it makes us breathe. Not for nothing in many philosophies is the fundamental force behind life seen to be the breath. Vigorous breathing increases yang. In yoga the bellows breath increases our metabolic rate – but it's hard work! Taking exercise, or vigorous physical work, is often easier and more natural.

Any exercise that does this is good. Walking as fast as possible for brief periods makes you breathe deeply and gets you warm. Running is better, but not to exhaustion and not so that you grow too thin. If you are already thin, then some form of resistance training is beneficial, to encourage muscle growth and create more yin 'bulk'.

If being thin is not your problem, resistance training is still beneficial as it tones your muscles and makes it easier to climb stairs and run for buses successfully!

Keeping active in general is beneficial. This means cherishing your individuality as long as possible, and in particular your independence from assistance. Learn to cook for yourself or your friends, go shopping (not just online!), get out and meet people. If your finances, hearing and eyesight allow, go to shows and performances.

In short, don't just sit around and watch television or films at home.

Your local neighbourhood probably has many features that your community has no resources to maintain. A local stream or river that needs cleaning perhaps, pavements that fill with litter or branches; a statue fouled by birds; a meeting hall that needs to be painted. Try to take an area and keep it clean so that life can flow along it – otherwise, yin easily takes over, in the form of accumulations of rubbish, dust, leaves, water and earth.

Help neighbours, even if younger than you.

Mentally, meet people and talk, even argue. Do things together. Read, reflect, write to newspapers with your comments. To some extent, make a nuisance of yourself. Write a blog and read others' blogs, but avoid too much sitting around, even writing at a computer.

If you spend much time at a computer, make sure to take regular breaks during which you get up and move around for a few minutes. Foster yang!

Stimulation

Yang is the fizz that makes the world go round – our motivation to strive:

• The politician whose emotion sways our opinion

- The music that transports us
- The advertisement that persuades us
- The images that excite us
- The affair that kindles our ardour
- The party that animates us
- The research and development that leads to more wealth through jobs and products
- The achievement that inspires us
- The preacher who makes our soul yearn for better things

We like this feeling: it stimulates us! We often want more of it! However, it is not all good:

- What do we think of people swayed by every political issue, their votes too easily influenced?
- What of the party-goer who just parties and sleeps?
- What, of the lover who always seeks new pastures?
- What, of the individual who continues the excitement via drugs?

We think of these people as lacking direction and, probably, of being selfish.

Boosting the yang state of mental excitement with drugs or other artificial means may be essential for short periods under extreme circumstances, as in war or times of peril, but it depletes our yin resources quickly. We then take a long time to recover.

Even coffee, which for yang deficient people is often a boon, may easily over-stimulate and exhaust us. For days after we may lack bounce, especially if we are also yin deficient[5].

5. http://www.acupuncture-points.org/yin-deficiency.html

The sun at first warms then tans us but too much of it burns us.

Overgrowth is a sign of excess yang exhausting yin. People become frayed out, lose their resilience, are wasted. Some people grow too fast too early and it may take many years, even into old age, before their yin catches up with their yang and they feel confident in themselves and their bodies. In the meantime, their enthusiasms are hard to control and their bodies are too thin or yin deficient. Usually they are more prone to disease and they need more sleep than they think they need. They often have large appetites but the food eaten is not reflected in more flesh unless they take care to chew and digest it well, and exercise, especially with resistance training to build muscle, strength and endurance.

Stimulants that over-boost yang

A man rang me from abroad asking what to do when he had self-administered huge amounts of electrical and drug stimulation including electro-acupuncture and amphetamines. The first effect was, at expected, increased alertness and energy. Those primary effects then proceeded to hyperventilation, high blood pressure, a racing heart-beat and feeling 'wired' all the time, as if he was taking huge doses of strong coffee every few minutes. His hands shook, he could not concentrate, he felt restless and exhausted. He was unable to sleep. He thought he was going 'mad', living a hyper-active nightmare. His speech was rapid and somewhat incoherent. He said he dared not stop all his stimulants as he feared that his heart would stop.

Here was a case of excess yang stimulation that had all but exhausted his yin resources. When, after considerable persuasion, he did stop his stimulants he entered a long phase of the secondary[6] effects of his self-treatment – inertia and low spirits:

6. http://www.acupuncture-points.org/primary-and-secondary-actions.html

yang deficiency – but in his case by then he also had symptoms of yin deficiency.

Excitement is not always beneficial: my children entreated us to let them watch horror films late at night. They loved the excitement. But the next day they were irritable and exhausted.

Inspiration

Yang factors that may inspire us include philosophy, politics, music, art, wit and humour. All of these, you may notice, are often suppressed or controlled by society and its government as yin factors become stronger and it fears change.

Samuel Hahnemann wrote his major treatise on homoeopathy, the Organon, starting around 1795 with its last – 6th – edition not published until 1921, long after he died in 1843.

Homoeopathy must be one of the most yang forms of treatment conceivable, being apparently without form or substance, based on a concept of stimulation rather than suppression of existing symptoms, and with no currently understood, acceptable or provable mode of action. It is consequently condemned by practical science: yet capable of transforming health.

Aware that the homoeopathic medicine, known as the 'remedy', seemed 'weak' when compared to ordinary medicines, he wrote – as a note to Organon paragraph 259 – that 'in the quiet of the night, the soft tones of a distant flute inspire feelings of bliss, but are inaudible amid the clamour and noise of the day.'

So: control the level of stimulation!

Heat and Encouragement

As yin needs yang for its warmth, inspiration and drive, yang needs yin for rest and recuperation.

A plant needs earth to grow up through. The lily on the pond surface with its beautiful flowers starts down in the mud at the bottom of the pool and pushes up towards the light through the waste matter and water.

Without a supportive and shepherding family or community to grow up in, the yang energy of youth loses its way.

It becomes easily misled and unstable, prone to (self-)destructive wilfulness.

Without good food, the flesh and muscles don't fill out with youthful lustre.

Without love and nurture, the spirit develops fitfully, selfishly, wastefully.

Without educational guidance and limits, the yang lacks direction and self-awareness, and wants for the skills it needs to understand, explore and exploit the world.

Encouragement

As we grow we need the sun. Most children crave encouragement and praise from their parents and many teaching methods use this to help students reach targets.

Plants need sunlight for the energy it gives them.

The sunlight also stimulates the plants photo-receptors to start germination and growth of leaves, then the formation of buds and eventually flowers and seeds.

Without that light, or equivalent source of energy, plant growth is retarded.

Plants without sun grow more slowly, if at all. Often they are stunted: they lack resilience and their flowers may not go on to fruit or seed. They lack yang.

Animals given too little sunlight tend to move more slowly.

People in high latitude climates where the sun is low in the sky for long periods can suffer from depression.

Everyone, especially the young, benefits from encouragement, from love and attention.

Animals not given this fail to grow up properly and mentally and physically they don't mature. In turn, they don't give love and encouragement to their offspring, so the pattern continues down the generations.

A lack of encouragement (ie yang deficiency) can become the heavy hand of repression (excess of yin) stifling self-expression and making the child withdrawn and depressed. Later it will lack confidence and be unable to achieve the success it might have gained.

So: make sure you give warmth, encouragement, friendship and support to people when you are well. (Not least because, perhaps when you in turn need it, you will have friends or a community in place to return the favour.)

Especially do this for the young, whether they be children or beginners or new enterprises.

Sunlight

The sun is our largest source of yang energy. Regular exposure fosters yang energy and helps to chase away the effects of cold, damp and wet. People with fair skin or red hair should take more care, but they still benefit from the sun. It benefits us physically and mentally.

Even in winter, the sun's light is beneficial, so get out and walk in it. In very high latitudes or in winter your skin makes little or no Vitamin D, but your body is highly adaptive and the light itself is beneficial.

The action of walking (or exercising in the daylight, if not sunlight) benefits your yang energy. Don't overlook the importance of natural light, including sunlight, on the health of your eyes and brain. (For example, we now know that sunlight, even if weak, stimulates our brains to produce serotonin, which aids sleep, and controls melatonin, benefiting fertility.)

Exercising vigorously in itself is yang promoting, and in sunlight is even better.

However, like all things yang, too much strong sunlight is destructive. Sunburn affects old and young. At maturity we can usually manage it better, partly through taking precautions and partly because our bodies are stronger than when young.

As you age, your yin resources deplete, so ration your sunlight accordingly.

Too much sun overheats, dries and burns us, a fact exploited now by a huge industry.

If your health is dominated by Damp and Cold, if possible take regular breaks in places that are warm and dry, and dominated by the colours of red, yellow and orange. For more on why, see the section on Fire in the chapter on Yin, Yang and Matters of State.

So: avoid cold and damp and seek to maintain warmth. Welcome exposure to the sun.

One more thing!

Independence

A further aspect of yang deficiency is that of lack of independence, showing as deficiency of:

- courage
- self-defence
- decisiveness
- clarity of thinking
- dynamism
- creativity

Treatment for this in Chinese medicine often includes treatment for the Gallbladder[7].

7. http://www.acupuncture-points.org/gallbladder-deficiency.html

CHAPTER 10

Dangers of Excess Yang

This book is about yang *deficiency*, but what happens when you get **excess** yang?

Too much yang is destructive, just as too much yin is suffocative. If not managed (a yin word) yang can run out of control.

For example, the human world is currently subject to many acts of terrorism. This is an example of yin reaching its culmination then turning into yang. Were that yang force to win, later on you would then see the opposite occurring, where a yang force runs out of inspiration and becomes domineering and tyrannical.

Islam has inspired strong reactions, from the humdrum conformity of Western life back towards strict Sharia law. Sharia is also a way of life that controls yang energies. Too strict, and it produces its own breakaway forces.

Christianity has inspired war in the name of God. Many of its sects, while initially inspirational, became controlling and tyrannical.

Communism inspired struggle and overthrow of oppression, but then became regulatory and repressive of initiative and enterprise.

For terrorists wishing to overthrow the state, ends justify

means: the murder of innocent participants and slaughter of democratically-minded opponents.

Young people want to travel and explore. If allowed to, they move on and mature. If prevented, that need may fester, leading to acts of destruction, some self-inflicted.

Young people, sometimes naïve, are attracted by the romance of armed struggle against repression.

I would guess that some of those so attracted did not much play competitive sports in their youth and before their maturity, and/or were over-controlled by parents who wished for nothing but the best for their children, over-schooling them, ensuring their safety, trying to protect them from the perceived dangers of multi-culturism and alien ideas, and encouraging careers in safe, conforming professions.

The point is not that these religious ideas are or were right or wrong, because your individual point of view decides that, eventually to be supported or condemned by history and philosophy, but that the energetic imbalance grows too strong in the direction either of yin or of yang.

When yang is (comparatively) deficient only as a result of yin excess (control), yin will tend to want to become ever stronger for fear of yang 'break-out'. Eventually, however, yang will still break out and may then transform the situation or, worse, destroy the status quo.

When yin is not excess but yang is deficient, then yang ideas can inspire the actions that mend the balance between them.

- The bored schoolboy, aimlessly gaming, suddenly sees the girl outside that inspires him to the chase, incidentally improving him in many ways, such as to clean and present himself better.

- The girl, shy about her body, sees in the media what she can become, and is inspired to eat and exercise better.

- The professional architect, lawyer, accountant or builder, successful but unfulfilled, is inspired by a philosophy of life or religion to re-train and transform into the healer, writer, osteopath or priest.

- Of course, if the healer cannot make ends meet or is crushed by the demands made upon her, she may be inspired to re-train and become the builder or gardener, lawyer or accountant.

When yang is deficient, seek the idea that stirs change. Ideas are the most yang things possible. (They can, however, act for good or bad, but as mentioned at the beginning of this book, yin and yang carry no moral baggage. For example, 'All You Need is Love' was a great song and inspiration in 1960s, strongly Yang in nature. 50 years later, that song had become part of a tradition – Yin-like. New generations seek new, different, chants and some people will be as influenced by the new songs as their grandparents were by the Beatles. The old chants were not more right or wrong than the new ones. Just different.)

Yang Excess

If you were to increase your yang energy so much that it became excessive, at least in relation to your yin energy, what might happen?

These are the kind of symptoms you might suffer:

- Over-reaction, or reactions that are too fast for either your or other's comfort. This can occur in terms of personality, making you pushy, demanding, triumphalist and quick to anger, or in terms of your body, making some functions process faster than others.

- For example, you might find that your small intestine pushes your bowel contents through to your large intestine faster than the latter can take it forward. This leads to clumping in your lower right abdomen, with symptoms like irritable bowel syndrome.

- Another example is when you find you get very strong tension arising before an event, making you tongue-tied and awkward, perhaps with a headache.

Here are some of the other symptoms you might experience:

- Waking too early; insomnia
- Excessive or irregular perspiration
- Palpitations of the heart
- Dryness of membranes and skin
- Bitter taste
- Thirst
- Diarrhoea and offensive smelling stools
- Emotional disarray, leading to physical symptoms such as headache
- Red eyes
- Tendency to feeling hot, even feverish
- Angry outbursts in over-reaction to events and people: road rage, for example.
- Hysterical laughter in reaction to life.

In Chinese medicine, dealing with this takes two forms, equally important.

1. Clear, calm, cool or dissipate the excess yang
2. Regulate yin to absorb and control yang

There are many ways to achieve success in this, including counselling, education, behavioural therapy, diet, acupuncture, massage, games, exercise and herbs.

CHAPTER 11

Treatment

Your body is yin compared to your mind. You may be yang deficient, but to live you require a body. In Western and Greek mythology, matters of spirit were praised, those of the lower physical energies were feared and criticized.

In Christian thought, those of the body could become temptations that led you to Hell.

In the I Ching, for life, both were needed and neither criticised.

So: to strengthen yang energy, find ways to harmonise yourself with your baser energies and desires, to use their power and wisdom to ground yourself.

You would expect Chinese medicine to have remedies for yang deficiency. It does. But, even so, practitioners look at a wider picture than just yang deficiency, which may form only a part of a full Traditional Chinese Medicine (TCM) diagnosis.

Those other parts of the diagnosis may suggest clues to the cause of the yang deficiency.

TCM's ways of treatment cover many modalities.

- Interacting, talking and encouraging may be as important as information and education. The interactions help to encourage the patient to participate more, to play a little, to enjoy humour and the company of the practitioner – all yang energy attributes.

- Back this up with herbs[1] that, for example, strengthen the digestion and gently nudge the patient's metabolism to become more relaxed and able to manifest yang qualities.

- Use acupuncture[2] to clear pain and stagnation, to balance the different zang-fu[3] energies so that they function in support of one another and to keep Qi moving smoothly along the channels.

- Moxibustion[4] on specific acupuncture points or areas helps the patient's energy to move away from cool to warm.

- Touch and massage give physical encouragement, but they also have a spiritual dimension. Whether or not you believe in energy passing between people, the effect of touch is often steadying and strengthening. Someone who knows how and where to touch or massage has great power. With a knowledge of acupuncture theory and channels it can be healing.

- Advice on food[5] helps the patient to choose nutrition that suits his metabolism and then to eat the best way to increase his powers.

- Hot stones. Steam rooms and saunas also benefit yang, but should not be used for too long as they may drain yin, by making you perspire too much. If you suffer from a syndrome known as 'damp'[6], use them only for short periods. If you are also yin deficient[7], use steam rooms and saunas only for short periods.

1. http://www.acupuncture-points.org/chinese-herbs.html
2. http://www.acupuncture-points.org/acupuncture-medicine.html
3. http://www.acupuncture-points.org/zang-fu.html
4. http://www.acupuncture-points.org/moxibustion.html
5. http://www.acupuncture-points.org/nutrition.html
6. http://www.acupuncture-points.org/damp.html
7. http://www.acupuncture-points.org/yin-deficiency.html

- For long-term benefits, some people find talking therapy beneficial. Analytical and other kinds of psychologist who have themselves undertaken a journey of self-exploration may be able to help you.

- So may priests and shamans.

- Exercise – enough to get you out of breath – moves and distributes Qi, which leads the Blood to where it is needed. However, exercise should not exhaust you, and be careful not to get cold – to lose that vital heat you have built up.

- And on a lighter note, one more thing! Try cold showers – but! – there is a right and a wrong way to take cold showers[8]!

- I am suspicious of advice that you should just be positive and forever strive only upwards, ignoring the nether regions. Those nether regions may be sources of unresolved yang conflict: hidden away and contained, seemingly yin. If so, yang will break out sooner or later, a source of wonderful energy for you if channelled: hence, get help.

However, if a patient makes no changes in diet or lifestyle, all the treatment in the world will make little difference, as the condition will reassert itself.

To give an idea of how a particular symptom of yang deficiency might be approached, here is the thinking behind a diagnosis for cold hands.

Cold Hands – a possible diagnosis

Cold hands are often part of the yang deficiency picture (though having cold hands can be due to other syndromes). The diagnosis is often that the coldness is because the energy in the upper part of the torso is defective, the upper part containing the Lungs, the Heart, and the Pericardium.

That the Heart and Pericardium are involved suggests that there may be an emotional problem, or a question over the

8. http://www.acupuncture-points.org/cold-showers.html

happiness of the individual, either now or at some time in the past.

Cold hands need warm blood to warm them up. The Heart circulates the blood and the blood will have good quality if the Liver has been able to store and replenish it overnight ... which needs deep restful sleep.

To produce blood in the first place requires the right food, a sound digestion and time to digest it. It also needs a spark to warm the digestion, which in Chinese medicine comes from the Kidney energy.

If the Blood[9] is to flow smoothly, there must be no Qi stagnation[10].

Qi Stagnation on its own could scupper the whole business, even if everything else is working well, because it would interfere with both Spleen and Heart energies, possibly Lung energy too. Helping the patient understand the effect of stress, diagnosed as Qi Stagnation, and work out how to deal with it, can be an important part of treatment. Also, there are acupuncture treatments for it.

Working with the patient, the importance of good nutrition would be emphasised, including eating at regular times and taking time to digest the food.

If this process of nutrition and digestion is good, the Spleen energy, supported by the Kidney energy will extract what is needed and send it into the blood stream to be taken to the Lungs and Heart.

Enough proper, restful sleep rejuvenates the blood. It then needs the Qi from the Lungs and movement from the Heart and the blood, now Blood (with a Capital B), goes to nourish and warm the hands. So, summarising what the patient can do for herself:

9. http://www.acupuncture-points.org/blood.html
10. http://www.acupuncture-points.org/qi-stagnation.html

- Sort out any frustrations or tensions, and organise life so that she is not over-stressed

- Choose the right foods

- Prepare and cook them, to be eaten warm

- Chew well, taking time

- Allow the digestion to do its work

- Make sure she sleeps well: this alone makes a huge difference

- Keep warm

- Exercise regularly, enough to get out of breath and warmed up

- Allow her lungs room and the space in her life to breathe. This means **good posture**[11] and regular activity that makes her pant, but does not exhaust her.

In terms of what an acupuncturist might do to help, after advice about diet, he or she would probably concentrate on treatment to improve digestion and sleep, and then discussing with the patient what sort of regular exercise or activity might be possible. He would also consider acupuncture points that stimulate yang energy, but might be cautious about using them until the treatment for sleep was effective.

---

11. Good posture alone makes a huge difference to the expression of healthy yang energy.

CHAPTER 12

Oppressed Yang – I Ching example

I have described various situations where deficient yang exists. Now for an example, analysed via a hexagram in the I Ching, the Book of Change.

The film Eye in the Sky[1] illustrates weak yang in the face of strong yin.

In this film, the War committee, chaired by the Alan Rickman character, is held back from taking a decision to strike known terrorists who are planning a major atrocity, by political views (yin) voiced by concerned ministers and others anxious to avoid hurt both to their own political position and to non-combatants.

They insist on referring up to higher levels of government (yin) for authority – all despite the desperate need for a quick decision voiced by the USA and in particular by the Helen Mirren character.

Equally, the individuals tasked with pressing the button on the strike missile are held back by pre-strike safety procedures (yin) which must be gone through rigorously before the strike button is pressed. (Incidentally, these individuals also have

1. https://en.wikipedia.org/wiki/Eye_in_the_Sky_(2015_film)

some yang-deficient signs of fear, and yin-deficient instability due to lack of experience.)

The yang energy, expressed forcibly by the Helen Mirren character, is weak by comparison with the yin-like safety and protective restrictions expressing the position of the individuals in the War committee. In fact, the strike is authorised only after she makes an unsafe, yang, decision to have the safety restrictions 'massaged', so that yang is justified and triumphs in the end.

This is what happens when a strong yang force is constrained for too long. Its weakness, in comparison to the prevailing yin energy, finds a way to express itself by some non-agreed route, often unpredictable.

Of course, the proposed terrorist action was also very yang: a suicide vest to kill many innocent people. This action was eventually prevented by the drone strike. But the film shows that the terrorists had to psyche themselves up first by engaging in a religious rite. The rite was yin, but the thought behind it was yang, derived from religious beliefs. The belief (yang) here was not enough. It needed a rite (yin) to give it strength and organisation.

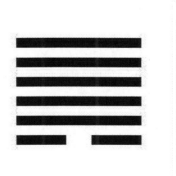

This situation is expressed quite well in hexagram 44 of the I

Ching. The bottom line, (known as the first line) is broken, or yin. All the other lines, above it, are unbroken, yang lines. This is an unstable position, with the lower trigram, representing *wind*, destabilising the situation.

This situation suggests that whatever action or inaction is taken, there is danger potential in the outcome: there is too much yang in the hexagram (5 yang lines supported by just one yin line).

To move on, urgent action is needed.

The lines suggest courses of action, ranging from

- the top line: "inaction", the result of which is a state of critical mass, and probably a breaking point in the existing structure ie a strengthening of the terrorist forces to the point when they destroy more of society. Changing this top line to a broken, yin line turns the hexagram into – "The Ridgepole Sags" – Hexagram 28.

- the fifth line (up from the bottom): suggests that maintaining and forcibly representing belief in the existing, 'stable and desirable' society with, dare one say it, firm indeed forcible education, leads eventually to "stability" – Hexagram 50. However, given the time limits of the story in the film, this would take too long.

- the fourth line: shows the danger of refusing to communicate with the other side and with elements in society that support it, leading to what the texts describe as 'misfortune'. If there is no such communication, only limited progress can be made, mostly "in small matters". Changing this fourth line to a broken line gives Hexagram 57. One text suggests that Hexagram 57 means resigning sovereign authority, an unacceptable outcome.

- the third line (up from the bottom) shows the results of

indecision – "Conflict" – Hexagram 6. So doing nothing gives no advantage.

- the second line suggests what happens if you merely protect your own borders: it suggests that you are retreating, or demonstrating "withdrawal" from the conflict – Hexagram 33.

- the bottom line: what happens if you change the bottom line from a broken yin line to an unbroken yang line? This makes all six lines into yang lines, forming Hexagram 1, the most yang hexagram of all, representing the Creative Principle, Yang itself. Changing this bottom line shows what will happen in any case, a very yang event ie an explosion. But there are two possibilities here, one being when the suicide bomber explodes herself in a crowd, killing many people. The other possibility, told in the film, shows the forces of 'good' destroying the bomber first – so there is still an explosion, but fewer people die. (Of course, that explosion starts a new cycle, whether caused by the terrorists or the forces of 'good'.)

These are my interpretations, and my choice of hexagram 44, not chosen by random methods but by consideration of the energies intrinsic to the story in the film. More situations can be considered by having two or more lines change at the same time, leading to other hexagrams.

In ancient times the Chinese used the I Ching to help understand the possibilities of different courses of action. It is still used by many people and not just in China. Members of the Chinese government may still use it. Those who use it claim that it leads them towards better decisions – better yang outcomes.

However, that does not mean such 'guided' decisions (yang word – decision) lead to perfection. They lead to what one hopes is the best, practicable solution for the time being, whether or not acceptable to everyone.

To use the I Ching requires a calm, contemplative state of mind and in my opinion should not be used hurriedly. For a good way to use it, requiring time and space which themselves incline you probably to greater understanding and more measured decisions, see the introduction to John Blofeld's edition[2].

2. I Ching The Book of Change by John Blofeld published first by George Allen & Unwin 1965

CHAPTER 13

With Weak Yang, What Else Happens?

Unless your yang deficiency was recent and of short duration, it will have become chronic. This means that your body is unable to improve much of its own accord in the normal way.

In other words, if you keep living and working without a change, your yang deficiency will continue, sometimes for years. But as explained, the more stable and long-lived your situation has been, the more sudden will be a change when it comes. So it is better to allow small changes to occur, or to incorporate change yourself.

Sometimes the right change is easy. It might be that you just need a relaxing holiday in a warm place during which you do nothing which might cause more yang deficiency (see the chapter 7 on the causes of yang deficiency).

For young people, an active – but not exhausting – holiday in even a cold place might be enough to stimulate the body to make the necessary improvement. For example, a skiing holiday is often very invigorating, though many young people return physically exhausted because they seldom sleep, partying through the nights almost as hard as they ski through the days.

But normally, you need to stay in a warm, dry environment, taking some exercise, not too strenuous and certainly not including standing for too long nor walking slowly nor carrying heavy things, because these deplete Kidney yang[1] and eventually jing-essence[2], the most deep-seated source of yang in your body.

You also need plenty of sleep and, for men, much less ejaculatory sex.

However, there is another factor to consider.

If your yang has been deficient for more than a short time, it will have also depleted your yin resources.

If you are more yang deficient than yin deficient, you might not notice the yin deficiency.

The yin deficiency, however, will show up in various ways, including

- restlessness,

- slight irritability or a short fuse,

- occasional flushes when not expected,

- poor sleep patterns,

- a sensation of heat, typically in your chest, palms or sole and,

- mild tinnitus,

- ... all possibly worse in the afternoon and early evening.

These are symptoms of mild yang excess due to yin deficiency[3].

Depending on how it manifests and which of your zang-fu[4] energy organs are most affected, you could find yourself sometimes unable to catch your breath properly, having to yawn but not always able to do so satisfactorily, occasionally short

1. http://www.acupuncture-points.org/kidney-yang-deficiency.html
2. http://www.acupuncture-points.org/jing-essence.html
3. http://www.acupuncture-points.org/yin-deficiency.html
4. http://www.acupuncture-points.org/zang-fu.html

of breath perhaps when talking or climbing stairs, your nose or ears suddenly feeling blocked as when descending fast from a height, and suffering from dryness of your skin or mucous membranes.

Why does this happen?

Remember that yin and yang are two sides of the same coin. If one is depleted, eventually it will deplete the other. They are just two aspects of the same thing – the Tao. Yang uses yin as its source of energy. Over-using yang depletes its supply.

When both are deficient, even if one is more deficient than the other, your body becomes less stable when adapting to life: you are more easily put 'out of sorts' and succumb to small irritations that normally would not be noticed. If you get ill, it takes much longer to recover and you may need treatment as well as a complete change of living pattern.

If yin deficient, getting hot may be a problem so a holiday in a warm country may be impossible: great for your yang deficiency, but it may worsen your yin deficiency!

And what about stimulants like coffee? For yang deficient people, an occasional coffee feels great. It bucks them up hugely. (Just the occasional coffee, mind!)

For yin deficient people, coffee stimulates their adrenal glands, which are already deficient. Initially they often feel better, but soon they start getting a sense of pressure in their heads, possibly with increased tinnitus. It makes them tense and unable to relax. Sleep may be affected, and during the days after taking the coffee(s) they may feel a slight 'tired' headache and general weariness.

Because of their yang deficiency they will feel cold, but because of their yin deficiency they will feel slightly 'bothered' and restless, more easily stressed, making proper rest and good sleep hard to achieve.

Another side to this is that yang takes a number of forms.

Weakening one form of it tends to weaken the others, but when there is also yin deficiency it becomes complicated.

For example, sexual energy and warmth are both yang. If, partly because of yin deficiency, there seems to be an excess of sexual energy – libido – the individual may want to wear less, if anything. Had yin been adequate, it would have absorbed the 'excess' yang, making the individual more energetic and balanced, so able to contain it. Without that balance, the situation is unstable.

Wearing less either flaunts sexuality or looks weird. It also makes you more susceptible to getting cold, inviting invasion of cold. Should it be a man and he ejaculates, he will now be both yin and yang deficient and will feel cold and tired.

The longer they persist in the individual's current living and working patterns the longer and worse these two deficiencies will become . Eventually he acquires clear signs of Kidney[5] deficiency.

These will have been put down to age, which in part they are, but in the absence of yin and yang deficiencies those ageing complaints might have taken many more years to manifest.

For instance,

- hearing suffers, not just from tinnitus but from deafness
- sleeping throughout a night becomes a distant memory
- anxiety and tension increase, requiring medication
- the need to urinate more frequently interrupts life
- the force behind urination weakens
- backache and aching joints – especially knees – become serious, requiring medication or surgery
- high blood pressure needs medication
- hair falls

5. http://www.acupuncture-points.org/kidney-syndromes.html

- skin dries out, needing moisturisers
- taste: you need more salt and pepper than before
- teeth and gums need more treatment
- concentration on tasks becomes harder
- memory issues become a problem
- in effect, you age faster

These are all signs of depleting Kidney energy as yin and yang become more deficient.

But Yang in Chinese thought represented Heaven: Yin was Earth. Man was made of Earth and stood upright on it, reaching upwards to Heaven, occupying the space between Heaven and Earth.

The spiritual dimension is vital to health. Whether this is represented by spiritedness (as distinct from spirituality) or by hope, inspiration, imagination, enterprise, a sense of a greater whole, or the Arts, drama, dance, music or creativity, all are yang forms of expression and necessary for spiritual health.

These forms of yang energy when balanced by healthy yin energy are reflected in a wholesome life.

PART II

THE WIDER CONTEXT

CHAPTER 14

Unpredictability and Yang Deficiency

As far as the body is concerned, the main signs of Yang deficiency have been explained. These are its ability to react, to defend itself, to adapt quickly and to keep warm.

If you are yang deficient, then by definition, comparatively speaking there is more yin than yang in your situation.

"It is the common fate of the indolent to see their rights become a prey to the active. The condition upon which God hath given liberty to man is eternal vigilance." (Atrib. John Philpot Curran)

You become increasingly yang deficient the more:

- You age (although most of us also become more yin deficient with age)

- Habits rule your life

- Certain are your beliefs

- Assured you are about your situation

- Comfortable you are

- Static you are

However, to compensate you need only a small measure of yang unpredictability – usually!

Children are yang. They are growing fast, itself a sign of yang energy; they have small yin bodies so easily show yang excess by over-heating and making noise. Because of having small yin bodies, they are restless and accident-prone; they are inquisitive, have short attention spans and need lots of food. Their presence is often disruptive, inconvenient, troublesome.

Wise grandparents benefit from having to look after them, because the children's yang energy can stimulate yang responses in the grandparent. This helps the grandparent remain alert and adaptable, mentally and physically. Of course, it also uses up the adult's yin resources, sometimes exhaustively.

What about you? Perhaps you go to the gym, every day at the same time. You do the same exercise regime. It's hard work. You get 'fit'.

The longer the period of time you've done this for, the more urgently you need to vary your routine. Ideally you change your regime a bit every week, testing your heart and muscles slightly differently each time. Or instead of always exercising only in the gym, instead run there and back, or over rough ground or over open country instead. Try different machines or weights. On some days do everything faster, perhaps with lighter weights. Or work with someone else who challenges you. If you go every day, don't. On some days spend the time examining the weeds outside your house.

If you never try interval training, try it. If you always do interval training, sometimes don't.

If you work sitting at a desk, try to stand sometimes to do the work. Take a walking break every 45 minutes – but change the interval occasionally. If your work is physical, be grateful for rests or for times when you have to sit to work.

If you are healthy, but eat the same foods every day, however 'healthy' they are, add the occasional garbage (hint – it's called junk food!). If you eat only junk food, you probably aren't reading this book.

If you always take the bus, try walking for part of the journey.

If you garden and only grow gladioli, plant the occasional cabbage.

If you always read the same newspaper, especially if it reflects your own views, occasionally read some of the others.

If you like solitary sports, sometimes try team or competitive sports. And vice versa.

Cultivate awareness of your situation and surroundings. Pickpockets and thieves are yang forces and benefit from absent-mindedness.

Overall, strive to be more independent and less dependent, or at least to maintain a balance between these two states.

Above all, do not trust your government or local council or community to keep you safe! They may do their best, but over-reliance on them is fatal, and is what often eventually happens if you live in a rich state that provides for its citizens as they age. If those ageing citizens rely on the state and its protection too much, they become susceptible to exploitation. They should cultivate scepticism and alertness.

If you are young, relying on the state for support does you no good. You will be healthier and probably wealthier in due course if you work to look after your own interests by earning an income and saving and investing your surplus, or starting a business. Failing that, take the initiative and build a network of friends to support one another in times of stress, for most surely those times will come as yang forces upset yin conditions and yin states run out of money.

What about Yang Environments?

Of course, if you live in a very yang environment, such as a war zone, you are more likely to be yin deficient due to your yang situation and its energy being at full pitch. You hardly need my advice to look for somewhere calmer and safer. Your quantity of yang energy is less than your environment's, or that of your enemy. Here, you must return to the essence of yang, that of retaining your identity by all means possible.

In hospitals, the accident, emergency and surgical wards are the most yang areas. If you work here, your life there will already be full of urgent decisions and unforeseen events. Your life needs more yin situations for its health.

In other parts of the hospital, where people are kept alive or convalesce, too much comfort and warmth may be bad: hospitals in the UK could at least reduce the air temperature to more normal levels to stimulate their patients' yang energy to keep themselves warm. Lower temperatures may also slow the advance of bacteria and viruses.

For health, avoid temperatures that are too cosseting: if the outside environment allows for it, open windows and turn down the central heating or air-conditioning a little.

Education, Research and Development

Since the most yang-favouring conditions arise from the mind, any state that ignores the spiritual dimension (whether or not religious), including the raising the 'spirits' of the people, could be accused of dereliction of its duty.

But beyond that it must concentrate on education, followed by measures to foster research and development.

Education: to help bolster this important yang quality of identity, should include awareness of the state, its history and culture and what it can, should and should not be expected to, provide; also understanding of other cultures.

Then research and development which are investments in the future. Money spent on them now delays gratification which means lower levels of state benefits provision until the benefits of R&D feed through into wealth, represented by infrastructure, goods and jobs.

The state should also urgently encourage initiative and enterprise and allow the winners to enjoy their profits, using them as good examples for others.

It should also attempt to inculcate respect for value. Today's world gives instant web access to untold knowledge and potential riches. Many expect all this for free, and become intolerant of paying for the work and investments by others, let alone their hoped-for profits. If Qi is to flow properly, then as valuable knowledge flows one way, payment in some form should flow the other way. After all, if we place no value on others' work – we want it for free! – why should others value what we do?

These aims are easier to accomplish, in principle, for younger, less-developed economies.

They are harder to implement in older, more developed countries, which have cultures of work and expectation that are often resistant to change, and have larger percentages of the retired, infirm or aged, dependent on the state for their health and living.

Blessed as we are with the internet, it has turned to be a very strong source of yang potential, but also of disruption and the spread of ideas that threaten the status quo – yin. All the more important to educate users in its benefits and dangers, to ensure we understand how to use it and how to protect ourselves and our devices (smartphones, hubs, homes, identities, computers etc.). That way yin can regulate it for general safety.

CHAPTER 15

What about Nation States?

A nation that ignores border protection may soon perish or be absorbed into a greater whole. This may be fine if there is a strong continuing culture and pride, as when Scotland joined the UK (Acts of Union 1706 and 1707 AD) — at least until the Scottish National Party arrived to allow grievances to air, and to strengthen the cultural identity with a view to the return of independence!

In a broader sense, if it wants to preserve its culture it must educate its children properly, and require immigrants to achieve familiarity with the country's culture, and some kind of allegiance to it.

Balance has somehow to be maintained between the yang and the yin energies. Here's a table describing a small selection of issues which lie under each classification.

Yang	Yin
Border Protection: defence	Culture
Patriotism	History
Idealism	Ritual
Aim to enrich oneself	Tradition
Profit Motive	Jobs and Wages

Aim to Enrich the Country	Living Standards
Immigrants and emigrants	Welfare and Health Provision
Self-interest	Compassion

The more stable and accepting of one another's cultures and ways of life that civilisations are, the less need be spent on defence.

But if neighbouring states have different cultures, more will or should be spent on defence.

If all the countries within a 'union' share the same political aims, they will need less barriers between them. Where any of the countries have different aims, they will need borders. For example, in the United States of America, each state has its own laws but all agree on the overall importance and political union of the country as a whole and support its Constitution.

Compare that with the European Union[1], where Great Britain was never happy with gradual progress towards political and fiscal union: its exit is perhaps eventually inevitable.

The contrary applies too, and is often overlooked when a long-lasting civilisation has many weak, ill, aged or needy citizens who cry out for health and care assistance. Money spent on this (yin-process) competes with money spent on defining and defending the country (yang).

There is an old (Royal) navy saying, 'One hand for the ship and one hand for yourself'. Applying this to nation states makes it plain that, in the absence of happy congeniality with its neighbours, a considerable percentage of the gross domestic product should be spent on border protection, security and preserving a clear sense of national identity.

This is not to denigrate immigration, because many immigrants will be coming to enrich themselves through work and enterprise, benefiting their adopted nation as they do so. They

1. [1] The European Union was set up not least to end the possibility of war between European nations, by forming a union which would be both political and fiscal, with free flow of people, services and goods.

are yang forces that an old or complacent country may really benefit from. But if immigrants become too yang, they can become destructive. So the nation must educate them in its cultural heritage and, this theory suggests, demand their allegiance.

Border awareness includes combating the dangers of cyberterrorism.

Applying a few of the other concepts in Chinese medicine, such as Damp[2], Phlegm[3] and Qi Stagnation[4] one can see that Damp and Phlegm may be represented by low levels of individual health, understanding, education, awareness and tolerance, with too great a reliance on the State by many including the aged, infirm and unemployed or unemployable. Damp and phlegm in the form of mist and fog obscure the real needs of the state from view, over-emphasising the needs of the many.

Qi stagnation might be poor infrastructure and communications, and resistance to change caused by over-regulation, health and safety provisions and legal protection. These stand in the way of the adaptation by the body politic to the creation of more yang energy.

In a broader sense, it means trying to keep yin and yang in balance. If a country is always in debt, unable to pay its way, eventually its creditors will reduce their business with it. Either that, or the country's currency is devalued, making imports more expensive and exports cheaper. That automatically lowers the standard of living and makes the country's labour force cheaper for outsiders, so eventually business picks up and after a period of comparative poverty, wealth begins to return to the country. (That assumes that the country allows the forces of yin and yang to interact smoothly. If it imposes controls, yang forces for profit will be retarded and the country will take longer to get on its feet again.)

2. http://www.acupuncture-points.org/damp.html
3. http://www.acupuncture-points.org/phlegm.html
4. http://www.acupuncture-points.org/qi-stagnation.html

A stable society easily becomes too yin. Accepting immigrants who are young, energetic, fit, hard-working and able is highly beneficial, bringing as they do, creative and enterprising yang energy with them to the state. Allowing the aged and infirm to move abroad may help to reduce yin 'drag'.

But those older members of society embody the country's traditions and stability, so losing too many of them leads to volatility and insecurity.

Dictatorships and totalitarian states can last surprisingly long when they excel in repression, though as history demonstrates, no such state lasts forever. But democracies, if their amenability to new ideas and change is not suppressed, have a comparatively greater chance to survive as such for longer, whereas dictatorships tend to fail after a few generations.

A nation where any sector or class becomes either too powerful or too weak is also open to sudden upset. For a country's health, it must be possible for people at low levels of society, through imagination, energy, vision and drive – and education – to move up through the classes. It must also be possible for those in the 'favoured' classes, through indolence, ignorance, feebleness or misguidance to sink down.

Any ongoing supposedly stable situation lulls us into a false sense of security. Just as walkers immersed in their cell phones are a danger both to others and themselves, so a country can proceed to its own destruction by not remaining alert.

That yang alertness and awareness is the prime requirement for ongoing health in this broader sense.

However, maintaining a strong yang state of alertness is not comfortable. Sparta was a small nation besides Greece but maintained a highly yang fighting force which made it militarily fearsome and dangerous. Even today the word 'spartan' shows how economical were their yin qualities.

The Vote

In a healthy democracy, periodically the people (yin) vote for who shall represent them or become their leaders (yang). This vote is the occasion when, acting as one, the people's action is yang and the would-be leaders, having made their pitches, are dependent (yin). Then, until the next vote, the leaders are yang again. (Of course, if the leaders act intolerably, the people can rebel. This produces a very yang situation of instability and potentially violence, as such leaders seldom go quietly.)

Educating the people on what to look for in leaders is therefore important, as is getting them to vote. That voters will accept the blame for disasters occasioned by the actions they voted for may be too much to expect.

CHAPTER 16

Using yang safely

Eventually, after taking the advice in this book you will expect your yang energy to revive!

You may think that yang energy is always disruptive, unpredictable, over-heating etc.: inspirational perhaps, but possibly 'unsafe'!?

Not at all! But for it to manifest safely, it needs to combine with yin energy, pushing the latter to achieve more.

Yang and Yin are two sides of the same coin. Too much of either is unbalancing. The best way to get yang energy to benefit you or your environment is often first to develop yin resources that you can draw on.

In other words, start small. Here is what you might do if you are in business.

First, build yin resources:

- Look into whether there will be a market or demand for what you want to do.

- Investigate your likely needs, drawing on past experience, teaching and people's knowhow. This is your R&D: research and development phase.

- Save. The savings may be in terms of health – in other words, rest, eat well, exercise, a loving environment ...

- ... or they may be financial, in terms of putting money aside, or building a business that produces an income you can rely on. Saving means delayed gratification.

- Acquire the ability, or people, you will need, and train them.

- This rest-time also allows yang energy to recover.

Then, using your resources, start in a small way to build, deploying yang.

- Provide (yang) inspiration for the people (yin) you employ or lead

- Give them something to look forward to

- Set targets to aim for

- Explain rewards to expect

- Reassure them of your support

Of course, if you are in business, you may mount a surprise attack, even a hostile takeover, to outflank, weaken or buy out your competitors. Very yang! But that requires considerable yin resources, is disruptive and may shake things up too much for comfort. It may also make enemies that impede your progress later.

Then, starting small, build systematically.

Done this way, you enter the market surreptitiously, almost unnoticed, and frequently ignored by others. As you build, they only notice you when it is too late, by when you are out-competing them and already own part of the market.

This way, also, you can more easily adapt to the new market you have moved into. Its needs may be slightly different to what you had expected.

Had you swept in with your own agenda, you might have overlooked vital information and market needs that are harder to re-organise your business around once you have already made big investments.

Examples of this approach are many:

- The street-trader who builds the empire. Eg, Marks and Spencer; Philip Green, Richard Branson.

- The foreign company that starts small in a new country, disregarded at first. In the United Kingdom, this might be Aldi or Lidl, supermarket chains that were well placed to take advantage of financial woes starting in 2008.

- The business that starts in someone's back bedroom or garage: Apple, YouTube, Ebay.

- The body-builder who came from nowhere to take over the market. Charles Atlas, Arnold Schwarzenegger

CHAPTER 17

Yin, Yang and the Movement of Qi

Health, of an individual or a country, or indeed a world, does not mean total security. A secure state can nourish its youth more easily, but if security is too strong it will inhibit movement of ideas, goods and people, which leads to a build-up of yang frustration.

Health works when there is a steady flow between yin and yang states of existence.

The more powerful and stable a society or state, the more it lays itself open to a yang disturbance and the more it strives to guard against it. Modern life produced the internet. This boon brings information and danger as yang forces of imagination and mischief seek to undermine otherwise stable yin situations.

Why do hackers hack? Lots of reasons, pretty well all classifiable as yang responses to yin conditions. As people age, their yang mostly reduces and they become more conservative. Youth, usually more yang, keeps destroying the bubble of security that every generation works towards.

We put money aside for retirement in the form of savings, property, pensions: assets. The state demands its share of your income and savings, to preserve itself, its infrastructure and well-being. You work to protect your own. If the state gives back enough in value to match your contribution, you are probably happy. If you don't get enough, frustration builds and you begin to get Qi Stagnation[1].

Qi Stagnation is yang seeking release.

What about those few who will not work, though able to do so? Initially the state supports them, but eventually it reduces or limits their income and living standards. If it does not, then one portion of the population ends up supporting another part of the population, indefinitely. This produces victimised and aggrieved states of mind, never healthy, because one part of the population always expects to receive, never to give[2].

For health, a continuous giving and receiving should occur.

Damp in the countryside

In **countries** where yin forces prevail, you see what happens when the land is flooded. Everything slows down, areas cannot be reached, lives and properties are lost: clearing it up is hard work and time-consuming. It takes time before life begins to proceed normally again.

For the country this is economically costly. (This might be equivalent, in Traditional Chinese medical terms, to Spleen[3] deficiency leading to Damp[4] and possibly Phlegm[5], causing stagnation of Qi and unclear decisions from the Gall-bladder[6]!)

In terms of policy, thinking becomes confused and too many

1. www.acupuncture-points.org/qi-stagnation.html
2. This happened in Belgium, where the Flemish have historically been forced to support the Walloons when the latters' living standards were threatened as their industrial and mining base collapsed. The Flemish have, not surprisingly, tried to emancipate themselves but the Belgian constitution prevents them from forming a political party of their own. See 'A Throne in Brussels' by Paul Belien, Imprint Academic 2005.
3. http://www.acupuncture-points.org/spleen.html
4. http://www.acupuncture-points.org/damp.html
5. http://www.acupuncture-points.org/phlegm.html
6. http://www.acupuncture-points.org/gallbladder.html

undecided or ill-decided matters take up the government's time, when a firm decision, early, might have avoided them: 'a stitch in time saves nine!'

Statecraft, to succeed, must protect and maintain the state as a whole. If too many resources are spent on behalf of one or more strata of society, no matter how needy, to the detriment of the preserving the state as a whole, the state may collapse: a mess! (Mess – very yin word, requiring yang to sort it out!)

As a state tightens its grip, it imposes conditions that can become, in effect, damp-like.

To increase safety and to reduce deaths on the roads, the speed limit is decreased. Things happen more slowly, and there may be a deadening effect on the economy. Of course, the state reserves the right to break the rules, as with the Fire services, the Police and the armed forces. But for the rest of society, the speed limit is a damper on free and easy movement.

To stop the rich enjoying their wealth, tax limits are imposed. These are applauded by those who favour strong state – yin – control and demand more equality, but unless the state stops people emigrating (as demonstrated in many countries over many years) enterprising yang individuals will flee to more amenable countries. There they will be more able to create wealth through new products and jobs.

East Germany has taken decades to overcome 45 years of communist control. Somehow it failed to produce the yang individuals who, for example, in Poland – which had also lived under 45 years of communism – galvanized change.

Citizens who are not alert will not notice, or will willingly agree to these conditions. But the most yang individuals will end up either in gaol or abroad.

If a state does manage to control its people through tight management and conformity, it may yet be able to inspire them enough (through a process called brainwashing or education, often jingoism) to let it become a strong martial force. Here the state itself becomes very yang, which its neighbours perceive as threatening and warlike. Countries like this have included the Spartans, Great Britain at times, Germany before each of the two world wars, and North Korea in the early 21st century.

What happens if a country is also yin deficient?

This book is about yang deficiency, but because yang deficiency often accompanies, precedes or follows yin deficiency, what happens if a country is yin deficient?

You see what happens when a country is yin deficient at the end of a long and exhausting war. Whether it won or lost the war makes little difference to how yin deficiency manifests.

- Buildings, roads and railway infrastructure are wanting, often destroyed

- Lacking supplies, agriculture becomes more primitive, less able to supply the population: rationing and starvation become distinct possibilities, and the food available is very basic

- The means of communication, power supplies and organisation are meagre, needing urgent attention

- Lacking food, sanitation and dry buildings, people get ill more easily

- Without proper medication and hygiene, the health system is unable to cope with acute, infectious disease

- The health system fails to manage a wide range of chronic diseases so the weak, vulnerable and old die faster

- There are few, or only poorly paid jobs so people suffer poverty

- There are immense opportunities but no energy to exploit them, or the money or energy soon runs out

- People are tired and depressed, though if their country won the war, they may be more hopeful

Unfortunately, countries cannot take holidays. What happens is that either yang individuals find the means to start businesses, often black market ones – a yang response; or the victor helps, often by giving loans – a yin resource. With that help, enterprising yang leaders can start the rebuilding.

In either case, there has to be a yang inspiration that others (yin) can respond to. Then all you need is work, resources, and time (yin factors).

We saw a recent example in Greece which, at the time of writing this in 2015/16, had run out of money. It had no yin resources to fall back on, except in the form of borrowings. Greece was both lucky and unlucky. It had a strong resource in the yang spirit of the Greeks. They have a robust identity – yang. However, it has many islands and a long coast, a somewhat porous border, through which emigrants from the Middle East easily found their way. The Greek defence forces could not defend all their beaches against these massive incursions so their ability to defend themselves, the first requirement of yang, was weaker than it should have been.

The refugees increased the yin, the people in Greece, by thousands daily with consequent strain on yin resources, food, accommodation, care, healthcare etc. Their yang response was, first, to demand of the bigger yin, in this case the European union, that it absorb this mass migration.

Those immigrants who managed to be absorbed by the EU were likely to be mainly people with strong yang qualities: enterprise, energy, the desire to survive – to live, work and improve their lot – just what an ageing society needs – new life! But it takes time (yin) for these new members of society to find their feet, start work and build individual prosperity, so initially their presence yields little yang-type reward: at the start it draws on the yin resources of the adopted countries.

(One might add that, in the first place, Greece should not have become a member of the Eurozone, whether or not it was allowed to join the European Union. By voting recently to remain in the Eurozone, Greece tied itself to the rules of the Euro**zone**, which has financial penalties if a country fails to demonstrate financially viability. Had it left the Eurozone, Greece's currency could have fallen or risen to its natural level, allowing Greek businesses and the Greek economy to survive without the need for fines or strictures from the Eurozone countries. Maintaining your own currency is another way to protect your country.)

The same thing happened when East and West Germany united after the fall of the Berlin Wall. The East had been much weaker economically. Many of its young and able moved to the West part of the re-united country to make their fortunes, leaving in the East the slower, often older, more yin-type people and industries. It takes years, even decades, for the new yang energies to build up and bring prosperity to the new whole. Even in 2015, 26 years after the Berlin Wall fell, Germany's Eastern side lags its Western side economically.

Whether a country can or should welcome immigrants depends on circumstances. In the long run, it is nearly always beneficial. The migrants bring their energy and new ways of thinking, but in the short term, they impose a load on their new country, not often considered when people demand that their government accepts mass migrants. As local communities wake up to what will happen, they wonder where the money and resources are to be found to accommodate the influx.

That money doesn't come from the government! It comes from the people in the form of tax. A wealthy people can afford it even if they grumble. Less so a poorer country, but the theory of yin and yang shows that a poor country blessed by many yang individuals will become more prosperous, and faster, than a rich country populated mainly by yin individuals.

Factors influencing voters

In the 2016 referendum in the United Kingdom there were many factors on people's minds, but two main arguments: immigration and economics, the latter including freedom of movement of goods and people within the European Union.

Comparatively speaking these can be divided into yin and yang factors.

Yang	Yin
Freedom from constraint and Intolerance of control by others, in this case the perceived faceless bureaucracy of Brussels	Safety and Security as part of a greater whole: less likelihood of war
Power to be oneself, to define one's borders	Ease of movement of money, goods, agreements, people
Excitement at new beginnings	Continuation of familiar, stable conditions
Sense of victim-hood	Mutual support
Less responsibility for other countries	Rules and regulations shared with others for mutual benefit
Freedom to work individually	Benefits of solving problems together
Freedom to manifest whatever is perceived as one own's culture	Benefits of shared cultures
Less obligations	Sense of shared obligations

When planes are destroyed by terrorist atrocities, one sees clearly how security (yin) can never be 100% guaranteed when we also want the freedom (yang) to travel anywhere. Strong regulations, established to preserve health and safety in a community, irk those who wish to maintain or establish their own identity.

In terms of yin and yang and the movement of Qi between them, health does not include safety. It requires vigilance, both individually from citizens and from the State.

Qi Movement

Although this book is about Yang deficiency, more important still in the sphere of politics and trade is the smooth flow of Qi.

Qi is represented by people, ideas, goods, services and wealth as they move between and within nation states. If Qi circulates smoothly, yin and yang can re-balance each other.

When qi is prevented from circulating, either yin or yang will gradually predominate in a country, leading to frustration and tension, with one group suffering and another group succeeding.

Unless qi starts moving again, these differences will increase, making it harder for the hard-done-by to recover, and more envy and sense of injustice.

That leads to yin-type repression causing, comparatively, yang deficiency but eventually a build-up of potentially destructive yang pressure.

Tariffs are barriers to the smooth flow of Qi. Periods of protectionism have not for long, if at all, benefited global and individual country's economies.

Protectionism and trade barriers are put in place without understanding how energy flows. If energy can't flow, wealth cannot flow either and economies suffer.

There are many ways a country can retain its identity without the need for protectionism.

The next chapter looks at how Qi manifests according to the Five Elements, a philosophical concept probably as old as that of yin and yang.

CHAPTER 18

Yin, Yang in Matters of State

An ancient model is that of the Four Phases, also known as the theory of Five Elements.

The Elements are:

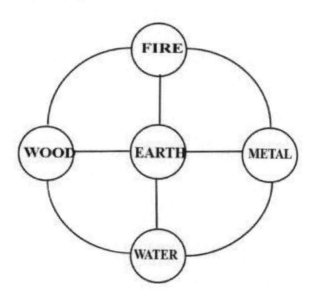

Water

The **Water** phase is the state between endings and beginnings. It has vast potential but not much that shows, like seeds waiting to germinate under the ground.

Winter, for example, comes under Water: the land lies barren, little grows, people rest (or at least, they did so in the past).

Night comes under Water, when we sleep.

Likewise, hibernation and re-training or re-equipping ourselves for the next stage.

The seed awakens but is not ready for growth.

In the body, this is conception and early pregnancy, very little sign of life yet.

Ideas are many, mostly un-elaborated.

This is the stage when one cycle of life is transformed into the next.

This is mainly yin in nature, formative and transformative through time.

This is a yin, waiting state.

Wood

Wood is the stage of growth, expansion, development, plans and actions. This has movement, usually upwards and outwards.

Spring occurs as the sun rises higher in the sky and things grow up towards its warmth.

Previously unformed ideas take shape and with the right decisions and actions grow into being.

Entrepreneurs love this stage. It's exciting and all-involving. Frustrations are obstacles to be overcome.

This stage includes the later stages of pregnancy and birth, infancy, childhood. Teenage years follow until self-awareness of position in society develops.

This is a yang increasing stage

Fire

Fire is when celebration of self develops. This is a fairly brief stage, though many try to prolong it.

Summer: the sun is high in the sky, leading to warmth or over-heating.

Full manifestation of the original idea or, its strengths and weaknesses are visible.

Your business is recognised – in the public eye.

The full beauty, energy and health of youth are apparent.

- Falling in love and Romance

- Parties and fun: celebrity culture

- Burnout and exhaustion

Fire is a yang state.

Metal

The **Metal** stage is when stock is taken, the benefits or results of the previous stages can be enjoyed and learned from, and better ways of doing things are appreciated or refined.

Things begin to decay and the seeds for the following cycle, whether in the form of health, wisdom, philosophy, teaching, or savings and investments, help to prolong or to cut short the life cycle.

Autumn: colder weather means we stay indoors or begin to wear more. Defensive actions are taken to ensure life continues.

Organisations become more static with received wisdom, rituals and an informed or regulatory culture tending to stifle growth, but also to steady it when the next Wood stage comes round.

The results of age are noticeable, for good or bad

A yin increasing state, the Metal phase gives way to the Water phase, renewing the cycle.

Earth

Earth is the ongoing and underlying life which is given expression by the other four elements. In the Five Element model its position in the cycle is put after Fire and before Metal, the idea being that after Summer comes the harvest, the waste products of which become the Metal phase.

Another ancient idea is that this Earth phase occurs briefly between each of the other stages, meaning that they either give Earth what it requires or receive from Earth their needs as they proceed.

I prefer the model shown above where Earth is, in effect, at the centre of the other four stages. (This has relevance in many ways in acupuncture where the so-called 'source' points of the main yin energies, those of Kidney, Liver, Heart and Lung, are Earth points. However, as mentioned above, both theories have merit and are used every day in clinical practice.)

Take the Earth phase as being the people, or the Earth itself.

If the people, then it is the resources and health they have to live.

For the successful, it is the good life. It is, unless they are in thrall to celebrity, what people aspire to, with enough wealth to enjoy life without needing to work.

For the unsuccessful, it is poverty.

For a nation, it is the grand mass of the people and their wealth.

It is the ongoing culture of a nation or family or company as it shifts, grows, is celebrated and refined or shrinks and dies or transforms through successive cycles of the four phases

Earth is yin, acted on by the other phases, but is their foundation and support.

The Yang States in the Five Element/Four Phase diagram

The yang stages of this are the Wood and Fire stages. The yin stages are those of Metal and Water. Earth, being yin and central, to some extent takes the form of the current stage. Each stage is influenced by its previous stage and in turn influences the next. In addition, each of the four stages has a balancing effect on its opposite in the cycle.

So, in health, Fire and Water phases balance one another; likewise, Wood and Metal phases.

This is particularly noticeable as between Metal and Wood, where Wood can move and shake Metal out of complacency, and Metal can provide experience and wisdom to steady Wood.

Metal also produces the inspiration, the ideas that eventually take shape in Wood.

But Water and Fire also have a major effect on one another. The Fire stage is what makes people in the early stages of a cycle, when they are in the Water phase, want to grow – their inspiration for all the work, whether in career or business, that leads them towards recognition and position in society.

Fire is controlled by Water in Chinese medicine theory: if not enough rest is taken, giving time for energy to recover in the Water phase, the Fire phase will burn dimly, splutter or burn out. The Water phase is also a constant reminder that Fire, for all its celebrity and fun, is transitory. Too much Fire or stimulation can exhaust resources, making rest impossible and diffusing power.

The movement of these phases can be seen in everything, from the universe to the life of a flea.

- Hitler, after the First World war (WW1 – very yang, Fire – destructive), after judgement (yin, Metal) went to prison (yin – Water). There he wrote a book 'Mein Kampf' which became the inspiration for the Wood phase that Germany entered in the 1930s, culminating in the Second World war (Fire). The energy expended in this war and the state of various nations and peoples after that war led to a long period of reflection (Metal) and then the (Water) recovery phase during which Germany nearly disappeared as a decision-maker, being occupied for many years by its victors. However, that period eventually led to tremendous potential, which manifested in industrial growth and strength (Wood phase) and its status as a major power and attraction (Fire), making a wealthy Earth for itself. Now, 70 years after its own destruction, many people fleeing war and hardship in their own countries wish to emigrate there. (Incidentally, this process displays Rule 4 qualities – see chapter 2.)

- In the Middle East, the countries mainly to the East of the Mediterranean Sea, wars have recently destroyed many lives. Yang ideas, mainly religious-inspired, have evolved out of long-term impasse, (eg enforced border definitions after WW1; Israeli-Palestine stand-off; unsuccessful completion of the invasion of Iraq and so on), and taken form and absorbed the energy of many young people attracted by extremism (Wood – often based on ancient and revered religious texts – Metal) leading to war and destruction (Fire) and the recognition, unwillingly, of the so-called Isil state. Next comes exterior pressure and ruin (Metal), to be followed by periods of recovery (Water). Should Isil succeed, then its (Metal) rituals will impose order for a while until the next cycle commences when yang again breaks forth.

- One could also argue that global warming has contributed. If the countries in that region had had sufficient water (yin), food would have grown more easily (Wood) and the desperation of many people to change their lives forcibly would not have taken root. Here the absence of yin (water) has led to an apparent yang excess (manifesting as religious-inspired war – Fire.)

- The business affairs of someone like Richard Branson go through similar stages. He started from a well-resourced family background. Being dyslexic may have been the making of him, meaning that others were needed to deal with the fine print (yin). That left him time to think and plan big – the Water phase (yin) leading to Wood (yang). Leaving school at 16 he formed Student magazine, later forming Virgin Records, initially to support the magazine. Since then he has continued to set up new businesses, some funding the next one (Wood). But he is also good at not being 'stuck' in the Wood phase. He enjoys publicity, knows how to use it (Fire) and makes sure that he is able to enjoy being celebrated (Fire) but also live a private life on his island in the West Indies (Earth). Not all his ventures succeeded: he had to sell Virgin Records in order to keep his airline, Virgin Atlantic, afloat. By living out of the public gaze when he needs to (Earth) he is able to reflect (Metal) and explore new ideas (Water). He is, apparently, often advised (Metal) not to start new projects, such as Virgin Railways! But so far he has mostly gone ahead anyway and succeeded.

- Each of Branson's businesses, indeed any business conceivable by anyone, will however go through the cycle. At some point after even great success every business must enter a Metal period of refinement or research and development (Metal and Water) or because of competition, disappear or be broken up or re-formed (Water).

- Deficient Yang also occurs where the previous cycle, when it reaches the Water phase, is unable to engender the ideas or resources needed for prosperous growth in the next cycle.

- Here either a longer period of rest, re-training and recovery is needed (Water), or help or advice from others must be sought (Metal). These can lead to better ideas (yang) and the means to put them into action (Wood).

Each of the four phases also has within it an internal version of the four phases. For example:

- As people age (Metal), they may start looking for meaning.
- That search comes about because they experience in some way a waste-land, the Water phase.
- From this emerges the Wood phase of experimentation, learning and discovery.
- At some point, they may be fortunate to enter a Fire phase of joy and greater Self-awareness.
- As a result, still later, they may find themselves in a deeper, more informed and possibly wiser position to aid others (Metal).

Possibly they may enjoy at the same time or later more cycles of the four phase diagram, as they develop new thinking, interests or hobbies, each of which has its own cycle.

To express one of the above ideas slightly differently, in assessing how yang situations occur, such as the current march of millions away from their home countries, it can be because a country's state is too yang for survival.

This can be because of war (Fire – Yang) and/or, as mentioned, because of yin deficiency (no water) – or a combination of the two.

However, those countries also have significant resources in their people and mineral deposits. Where these are combined, their country may prosper and be able to pay for the infrastructure (such as water resources) it needs. So another form of yin can to some extent make up for a deficit in water. (Just as inspiration (yang) can to some extent make up for tiredness, a form or yang deficiency.)

Global warming occurred we presume because we burned our yin resources (oil, coal, radioactive uranium) creating heat. If global warming does exist, it has characteristics of yin deficiency.

Normally yin deficiency is mended by rest and time, but yang ideas can produce inventions that, like drugs, appear to improve the situation. Let us hope for some good ideas: less yang deficiency!... and the entrepreneurs and right financial cradle to exploit them for our general benefit.

Imaginations, concepts and questions are among the most powerful expressions of yang.

They have immense power to influence and change us, but they have no physical form, unless articulated verbally or written down. Then they need work (yin) to manifest.

Most of our imaginations and beliefs are never given form, never articulated. As such they disappear, carried away in the maelstrom of our thoughts.

But those ideas that get the support of yin-work can change the world.

The person who asks the questions controls the situation.

Those who cannot imagine a better place, then explain what must be done to achieve it, and pose the questions that energise change, they and their countries may be, or are, yang deficient.

End of book request

Your Review?

Finally ...

Now you've read this book, *please review it!* As implied in the introduction, it aims to be not just informative, but *useful*.

If you think others would benefit from it, please post your opinion somewhere prospective readers might see it, such as on Amazon.

Here are links to the North American site (https://www.amazon.com) and the UK site (https://www.amazon.co.uk).

- Just click on the link above (either amazon.com or amazon.co.uk – or of course, your own country's equivalent)

- Put **"Yank Deficiency – Get Your Fire Burning"** in the search box at the top of the Amazon page

- When a picture of the book appears, click on where it says 'review' or 'reviews', then

- Click on "Write a customer review" and say what you think about it:

- You can give it 5 stars out of 5 – if you think it merits them, of course!

I hope you will be positive and constructive, but if you have major criticisms or reservations, I would like to know! Then I can improve it for the next reader.

Let me know through my website http://www.acupuncture-points.org on many pages of which there is a box for writing to me.

Thank you!

Appendix: Table of Food Energies

Table of Food Energies

The table below shows how Chinese medicine classifies many common foods in terms of their yin and yang qualities.

In some cases, you will see a food's energy occupying two columns, for example cooling **and** neutral, or neutral **and** warming. This means that the food may work in several ways, sometimes depending on its quality, provenance or season when picked.

Also, we are all different and it is possible that a food marked cooling might be cooling for me, but cold for you etc. In fact, a food might be described as cooling but in you act like a hot food. If you are unfamiliar with a particular food, add it to your diet gradually.

The word 'cooling' is also expressed in some texts as 'refreshing'.

Some foods may not be familiar to you and some (Western) foods have not been classified. Chinese medicine eventually classifies food, but it can take time.

What would happen if you ate nothing but warming or hot foods, as described in the tables? If you have skipped previous chapters to get here (!), it depends on your particular makeup, but many people would find themselves feeling hot and perspiring. That would be a short-term yang effect, but without 'yin' and 'Blood' foods there would be little long-term benefit to you.

Just eating hot or warming foods could have the following effects:

- Many people would find their stools became drier, more smelly and harder to pass

- Some people would get burning pains in the stomach

- Some might become shorter-tempered and less able to concentrate
- Some would get skin rashes or itches
- Body odour might become stronger
- Some would get urgent diarrhoea
- Eyes might become inflamed, red, itchy or dry
- Most would feel thirstier.

Please note: neither the author nor publisher accept any liability for results. See someone experienced or qualified if you are unsure what to eat.
#

Food	Nature	Cold	Cooling	Neutral	Warming	Hot
Abalone	yang			neutral	warming	
Alfalfa	Blood			neutral		
Almond	Blood			neutral		
Amaranth	yin		cooling	neutral		
Anise	yang				warming	
Apple	yin		cooling			
Apricot fruit	balance			neutral		
Apricot seed	yang				warming	
Arrowhead	yin	Cold				
Artichoke	yin		Cooling			
Asparagus	Blood		cooling	neutral		
Bamboo shoot	yin	cold				
banana	yin	cold				
barley	yin		Cooling			
Bean – mung	yin		cooling			
Bean – broadbean	balance			neutral		
Bean – sword bean	yang				warming	

Bean – kidney	balance		neutral	
Bean – string	balance		neutral	
Beancurd, tofu	yin	Cooling		
Bean -adzuki	balance		neutral	
Beef	balance		neutral	
Beetroot	balance		neutral	
Bitter gourd	yin	cold		
Black sesame seed	balance		neutral	
Broccoli	yin	cooling		
Brown Sugar	yang			warming
Buckwheat	yin	cooling		
Cabbage	balance		neutral	
Chinese cabbage	yin	cooling		
Peking cabbage	yin	cooling		
Caraway seed	yang			warming
Cardamon	yang			warming
Carp fish	yang		Neutral	warming
Carrot	balance		neutral	
Cashew nut	balance		neutral	
Cauliflower	yin	cooling	neutral	
Celery	yin	cooling		
Cheese – dairy cow	yin	cooling		
Cherry	yang			warming
Chestnut	yang			warming
Chicken	yang			warming
Chilli pepper	yang			hot
Chinese chives	yang			warming
Chives	yang			warming
Chive seed	yang			warming
Chrysanthemum	yin	cold		

Chrysanthemum – edible	yang		warming	
Cinnamon	yang		warming	hot
Clam	yin	Cold		
Clove	yang		warming	
Coconut milk	yin	cooling	neutral	
Coffee	yang		Warming	
Coix seed	yin	cooling		
Conch	yin	cooling		
Coriander	yang		Warming	
Corn (ie Maize)	balancing		neutral	
Crab	yin	cold		
Crab apple	balance		neutral	
Cream (dairy cow)	yin	cooling		
Cucumber	yin	cooling		
Cumin	yang		warming	
Cuttlefish	yin	cooling	neutral	
Dates	yang		neutral	warming
Dill seed	yang		warming	
Duck	balance	cooling	neutral	
Duck egg	yin	Cooling		
Eel – fresh water	yang		warming	
Egg white	yin	cooling		
Egg yolk	balance		neutral	
Eggplant (aubergine)	yin	cooling		
Fennel	yang		warming	
Fig	balance		neutral	
Frog	yin		neutral	
Fungus – black fungus	balance		neutral	
Fuzzy melon	balance		neutral	
Garlic	yang		warming	

Food	Nature	Cold	Cooling	Neutral	Warming	Hot
Ginger – fresh	yang				warming	
Ginger – dried	yang					hot
Ginseng -American	balance		cooling	neutral		
Ginseng – Renshen	yang				warming	
Goat's milk	yang				warming	
Goose	balance			neutral		
Goose egg	yang				warming	
Grapefruit	yin	cold				
Grapes	balance			neutral		
Green onion	yang				warming	
Hairtail fish	yang				warming	
Ham	yang				warming	
Honey	balance			neutral		
Horseradish	yang					hot
Iceland moss	Blood		cooling			
Irish moss	yin		cooling			
Jasmine	yang				warming	
Job's tears, coix	yin		cooling			
Kelp	Blood		cooling			
Kohlrabi	balance			neutral		
Kumquat	yang				warming	
Lamb	yang				warming	

\#

Food	Nature	Cold	Cooling	Neutral	Warming	Hot
Leaf mustard	yin		cooling			
Leeks	yang				warming	
Lemon	balance	cold	cooling			
Lettuce	yin	cold				
Indian lettuce	yin		cooling			

Lettuce root	yin		cooling		
Licorice root – raw	balance			neutral	
Lily bulb	yin		cooling		
Lily flower	yin		cooling		
Liver of pig	yang				warming
Loach	balance			neutral	
Lobster	yang				warming
Longan fruit	yang				warming
Loquat fruit	yin		cooling		
Lotus root	yin	cold			
Lotus seed	Balance			neutral	
Luffah fruit, loofah	yin		cooling		
Lychee fruit	yang				warming
Maltose	yang				warming
Mandarin orange	yin		cooling		
Mango	yin		cooling		
Marjoram	yin		cooling	neutral	
Microalgae	Blood			neutral	
Milk – cow	balance			neutral	
Millet	yin		cooling		
Mulberry	yin	cold			
Mushroom	yin		cooling		
Mushroom,tremelia	balance			neutral	
Muskmelon	yin		cooling		
Mussels	yang				warming
Mustard seed	yang				warming hot
Mutton	yang				warming
Nettle	Blood		cooling		
Nutmeg	yang				warming
Oats	Blood			neutral	warming

Food	Energy			
Olives	balance		neutral	
Onion	yang			warming
Orange	yin	cooling		
Osmanthus flower	yang			warming
Oyster	balance	cooling	neutral	
Papaya	yin	cooling	neutral	
Pea	yin	cooling		
Peach	yang		neutral	warming
Peanut unroasted	balance		neutral	
Peanut – roasted	yang			hot
Pears	yin	cooling		
Pepper – black	yang			hot
Peppercorn -Sichuan	yang		warming	
Peppermint	yang	cooling	neutral	
Persimmon	yin	cold		
Pig skin	yin	cooling		
Pig's bone marrow	yin	cold		
Pine nut	yang		warming	
Pineapple	yin	cooling		
Pistachio nut	balance		neutral	
Plums	balance		neutral	
Pollen from flowers	Blood	cooling	neutral	
Pomengranate	yang		warming	
Pomelo, shaddock or lusho fruit	yin	cold		
Pork	balance		neutral	
Potato	balance		neutral	
Preserved jellyfish	yin	cold		
Pumpkin	Balance		neutral	warming
Quail	balance		neutral	
Quinoa	balance		neutral	

Rabbit meat	yin		cooling		
Radish – Chinese	yin		cooling		
Radish leaf	balance			neutral	
Rasberry	yang		cooling		
Rhubarb	yin	cold			
Rice, glutinous	yang				warming
Rice, round-grained	balance			neutral	
Rock sugar	balance			neutral	
Root of Kudzu vine	yin	cold			
Rose bud	yang				warming
Rosemary	yang				warming
Rye	balance			neutral	
Sage	yin				warming
Salt	yin	cold			
Sea clams	yin	cold			
Sea cucumber	yang				warming
Sea eels	balance			neutral	
Sea shrimp	balance			neutral	
Seaweed	yin	cold	cooling		
Sesame oil	yin		cooling		
Shiitake mushroom	balance			neutral	
Shrimps, freshwater	yang				warming
Snails	yin	cold			
Soya sauce	yin	cold			
Soybean milk	balance		cooling	neutral	
Soybean oil	yang				hot
Soybeans	balance			neutral	
Spearmint	yang				warming
Spelt	balance		cooling	neutral	
Spinach	yin		cooling		

Spring onion	yang				warming	
Sprouts	yin	cold				
Squash	yang				warming	

\#

Food	Quality	Cold	Cooling	Neutral	Warming	Hot
Star anise	yang				warming	
Star fruit	yin	cold				
Strawberry	yin		cooling			
Sugar – molasses	yang				warming	
Sugar – white	balance			neutral		
Sugar cane	yin	cold				
Sunflower seed	balance			neutral	warming	
Sweet basil	yang				warming	
Sweet pepper	yang				warming	
Sweet potato	balance			neutral		
Sword bean	yang				warming	
Tangerine	yin		cooling			
Tangerine peel	yang				warming	
Tea (Indian and Chinese)	yin		cooling			
Thyme	yang				warming	
Tobacco	yang				warming	
Tofu, beancurd	yin		cooling			
Tomato	yin	cold				
Turnips	balance			neutral		
Vegetable oil	yang				warming	
Vegetables, green	Blood				warming	
Venison	yang				warming	
Vinegar	yang				warming	
Walnut	yang				warming	

Water caltrop	yin	cooling	
Water chestnut	yin	cold	
Water spinach	yin	cold	
Watercress	Blood	cold	neutral
Watermelon	yin	cold	
Wax gourd	yin	cooling	
Wheat	yin	cooling	
Wheatgrass	Blood	neutral	
Wild rice stem	yin	cold	
Wild yam	Blood	neutral	
Wine	yang		warming
Yogurt (dairy cow)	yin	cooling	

<<<<>>>>

Glossary of Terms

Blood http://www.acupuncture-points.org/blood.html An important concept in Chinese medicine, representing where our personalities have residence: people 'go to pieces' as they haemorrhage. 'Blood' is a form of Qi that is often called the 'mother' of Qi. In Blood deficiency, there is not merely poor memory and concentration but lack of confidence.

Channel or **meridian** http://www.acupuncture-points.org/acupuncture-meridians.html The presumed areas where qi flows: there are twelve primary channels but a large number of secondary channels, encompassing everywhere in the body.

Damp http://www.acupuncture-points.org/damp.html is a syndrome that causes swelling, heaviness and soreness.

Excess and deficiency http://www.acupuncture-points.org/excess-or-deficient.html are conditions that practitioners recognise because they often help decide on both treatment and advice for the patient.

Food Retention http://www.acupuncture-points.org/food-retention.html is a syndrome experience by overfed babies of all ages.

Heat http://www.acupuncture-points.org/Heat.html is a syndrome.

Jing-essence http://www.acupuncture-points.org/jing-essence.html The inherited genetic code's power, all too easily dissipated by bad habits and overstrain, but which gives us longevity and is our major underlying health resource.

Phlegm **http://www.acupuncture-points.org/ phlegm.html** is a syndrome with many symptoms, mental and physical.

Pulse diagnosis **http://www.acupuncture-points.org/ pulse-diagnosis.html** is a way to understand the health of the patient through taking the pulse.

Qi **http://www.acupuncture-points.org/qi.html** The energy of life and existence in all its forms, spiritual, mental, emotional and physical

Syndrome **http://www.acupuncture-points.org/syn-dromes.html** A disease pattern recognised in Chinese medicine. For example, 'Yang Deficiency' – the subject of this book, 'Heat in the Lung' – http://www.acupuncture-points.org/lung-heat.html, 'Blood Stasis' – http://www.acupuncture-points.org/ blood-stasis.html, 'Damp-heat in the Bladder' – http://www.acupuncture-points.org/bladder-damp-heat.html.

Tongue Diagnosis **http://www.acupuncture-points.org/ tongue-diagnosis.html** is a way to understand the health of the patient through observation of the tongue.

Wind **http://www.acupuncture-points.org/wind.html** is an important cause of disease in Chinese medicine.

Zangfu **http://www.acupuncture-points.org/zang-fu.html** The Chinese name for the 'energy organs'.

- 'Zang' are the yin organs (Heart http://www.acupuncture-points.org/heart.html, Spleen http://www.acupuncture-points.org/spleen.html, Lungs http://www.acupuncture-points.org/lungs-function.html, Kidneys http://www.acupuncture-points.org/kidney-function.html, Liver http://www.acupuncture-points.org/liver-functions.html, and Pericardium). Capital first letters indicate that the Zang is meant rather than the physical organ.

- 'Fu' are the yang organs (Small intestine, Stomach http://www.acupuncture-points.org/stomach.html, Large intestine, Bladder, Gallbladder http://www.acupuncture-points.org/gallbladder.html). Capital first letters indicate that the fu is meant rather than the physical organ.

- The term zang-fu means much more than the physical organ in question. For instance, the Bladder fu includes the various functioning activities of the Bladder in Chinese medicine, plus its channels and all the places influenced by them.

- Each zang or fu has its own functions and actions and, when the actions misbehave, syndromes (see above).

About the Author

Jonathan Clogstoun-Willmott is author of

Western Astrology and Chinese Medicine (1985)

Qi Stagnation (2013) = Book 1 in the Series Chinese Medicine in English

Yin Deficiency (2014) = Book 2 in the Series Chinese Medicine in English

Yang Deficiency (2016) = Book 3 in the Series Chinese Medicine in English (this book)

Yuck! Phlegm! (2017) = Book 4 in the Series Chinese Medicine in English

He maintains a website that aims to explain Chinese medicine in English:

http://www.acupuncture-points.org

He established the Edinburgh Natural Health Centre in 1983, having practised in London for several years before that.

He lives in Edinburgh, Scotland, Great Britain.

About the Publisher

http://www.frameofmindpublishing.com

Printed in Great Britain
by Amazon

16902190R00111